SPIRITUALITY IN
HOSPICE PALLIATIVE CARE

SUNY series in Religious Studies
Harold Coward, editor

Spirituality in Hospice Palliative Care

Edited by
Paul Bramadat,
Harold Coward,
and Kelli I. Stajduhar

Cover art by Susan Coward

Published by State University of New York Press, Albany

© 2013 State University of New York

All rights reserved

Printed in the United States of America

For information, contact State University of New York Press, Albany, NY
www.sunypress.edu

Production by Diane Ganeles
Marketing by Michael Campochiaro

Library of Congress Cataloging-in-Publication Data
Spirituality in hospice palliative care / edited by Paul Bramadat, Harold
Coward, and Kelli I. Stajduhar.
    pages cm. — (SUNY series in religious studies)
    Includes bibliographical references and index.
    ISBN 978-1-4384-4777-3 (alk. paper) — ISBN 978-1-4384-4778-0 (pbk. :
alk. paper) 1. Terminal care—Religious aspects. I. Bramadat, Paul
    R726.8.S627 2013
    616.02'9—dc23

                                    2012045684

10 9 8 7 6 5 4 3 2 1

Contents

Acknowledgments

THIS BOOK IS A joint project of the Centre for Studies in Religion and Society and the Centre on Aging at the University of Victoria, Canada. As many readers will know, it is intended to complement the analysis initiated in *Religious Understandings of a Good Death in Hospice Palliative Care*, also published by SUNY Press. While the formal religious requirements and sensibilities associated with a good death were significant concerns for the patients, family members, and hospice staff consulted for the first book, it was clear to the editors and authors of the first volume that the notion of "spirituality" was fundamentally changing the discourse associated with life and death in hospice care and, as such, would need separate and sustained treatment. Within contemporary health care settings, the increasing preference for spirituality instead of religion reflects processes unfolding throughout our society; nevertheless, the way these processes are transforming hospice palliative care is the focus of the current work. For this volume, we selected authors who could address the way the concept of spirituality is employed by patients, family members, hospice staff, and others in the health care system. Authors met in March 2011 to discuss first drafts of their chapters at a seminar held in Victoria and hosted by the Centre for Studies in Religion and Society. After this thorough process of peer evaluation, authors revised their chapters for this volume.

Funding for both volumes of this research was provided by the Canadian Institutes of Health Research. Special thanks are due to June Thomson for her assistance with library research, and Leslie Kenny (CSRS administrator) and Rina

Langford-Kimmett (CSRS secretary) for organizing the project meeting, managing the funding and editing process, and preparing the manuscript for publication. The artwork on the cover of the book is by Susan Coward, who is an artist, long-time hospice volunteer, and now a hospice nurse.

We would like to dedicate this book to Harold Coward, our friend and mentor who first conceived of the project, and to the tireless hospice staff who are always searching for better ways of knowing their patients and families—and themselves—during the dying process.

—PAUL BRAMADAT AND KELLI I. STAJDUHAR, COEDITORS
Victoria, British Columbia, December 2011

Introduction

PAUL BRAMADAT, HAROLD COWARD,
AND KELLI I. STAJDUHAR

IN TODAY'S WORLD, spiritual needs are experienced, expressed, and defined in a wide variety of ways. "Spirituality" may refer to a person's individual experience within a religious tradition such as Christianity or Buddhism. But more often than not these days, people do not feel their spiritual practices and beliefs need to be rooted definitively within a single or formal religious tradition. Others pursue ideas, beliefs, and practices they would call spiritual even though their approach to traditional religious questions (such as the existence of God, heaven, hell, and reincarnation) would be described as atheist or agnostic. It is arguably the case that one cannot effectively study contemporary religious life in North American and European societies without grappling with the increasingly well-defined cohort of "spiritual but not religious" people (not to mention the related groups of "spiritual but not necessarily religious" and "spiritual but definitely not religious" individuals).

In an earlier volume, *Religious Understandings of a Good Death in Hospice Palliative Care*, edited by Coward and Stajduhar (2012), the research team focused on the way those hospice patients and clinicians who are members of traditional religions understand the notion of a "good death." Setting out these traditional understandings was an important task. The current book focuses on the kinds of existential and spiritual questions posed within hospice palliative care contexts by persons

1

whose search for meaning has taken them beyond traditional religions such as Christianity, Islam, and Buddhism. For such persons—and they are, arguably, a rapidly growing cohort— "spirituality" is more important or more attractive than "religion." Such dying persons may describe themselves as atheists, agnostics, or in the increasingly popular terms of "spiritual but not religious" (SBNR) or "spiritual, definitely not religious" (SDNR). Some may define themselves as secular, humanists, or followers of New Age movements. However, regardless of the ways people disavow any formal links to or interest in a single religious perspective, many will still speak of spiritual needs as they approach their own deaths.

In this book, we acknowledge the difficulty of defining "spirituality." For our purposes, however, we suggest the following operational definition: "Spirituality" relates to an individual's pursuit of wholeness, well-being, transcendence, and oneness with the universe, whereas "religion" typically denotes an institutionalized system within which the individual's experiences are thought to unfold and be regulated. In discussions of spirituality in hospice palliative care, there is a tendency to contrast "spirituality" with the term "religious" in a way that frames religion as stifling the free development of spirituality by trapping it under dogma and tradition. The assumptions underlying this contrast are given careful critical analysis in chapter 1, "Hospice and the Politics of Spirituality." Also, to help in understanding the many ways the term spirituality is used in relation to hospice care, we include two personal essays by Patrick Grant and Elizabeth Causton, chapters 6 and 7 respectively. The intimate style of these chapters provides insights into persons who live outside of religious tradition yet feel it is worthwhile to share their experience of life and how they hope to be cared for when they are dying. But first, let us briefly retrace the developing use of the term spirituality within the founding of the hospice palliative care movement.

In the 1960s in London, England, Cicely Saunders introduced a new way of treating the terminally ill, which she called "hospice care." Saunders, a trained nurse, social worker, and medical doctor, held that humans should be able to die with dignity and at peace. This viewpoint originated from her

medical experience as well as her religious commitment as a
Christian. Saunders developed a program for care of the dying
based on three key principles: pain control, a family or community environment, and an engagement with the dying person's
most deeply rooted spirituality. Although the hospice movement began in a Christian context, it was clear from the start
that there was to be no "forcing of religion," and openness to
all religions and understandings of spirituality was encouraged.
While the first two of Saunders's principles have been well studied, the third, engagement with the dying person's most deeply
rooted spirituality, has been largely ignored in recent years. Our
first volume sought to fill that gap for religious people. This
second book is focused on those whose loyalty to a particular
religious framework or institutions is of no importance at all,
or of secondary importance to their individual spiritual journey.
The aim of both books is to help doctors, nurses, administrators, social workers, psychologists, chaplains, and volunteers in
hospice palliative care address the "spiritual pain" that often
parallels and accompanies "physical pain" in the care of dying
persons.

In Saunders's view, a good death honors the whole of
life—material affairs, human relationships, and spiritual needs
(2006, 266). She further defines a good death as "attention to
the achievements that a patient could still make in the face of
his physical deterioration and awareness of the spiritual dimension of his final search for meaning" (1981, ix). Spiritual needs
are defined by Saunders as follows: "'Spiritual' concerns the
spirit of higher moral qualities, especially as regarded in a religious aspect with beliefs and practices held to more or less
faithfully. But 'spiritual' also covers much more than that—the
meaning of life at its deepest levels as understood through our
patients' different religions." As Saunders puts it, "The realization that life is likely to end soon may well stimulate a desire to
put first things first and to reach out to what is seen as true and
valuable—and give rise to feelings of being unable or unworthy
to do so. There may be bitter anger at the unfairness of what is
happening, and at much of what has gone before, and above all
a desolate feeling of meaninglessness. Herein lies, I believe, the
essence of spiritual pain" (Saunders 1988, 218). In Saunders's

understanding, "spiritual pain" is parallel and interpenetrates with "physical pain." Indeed, Saunders coined the term "total pain" to take into account a broader conceptualization of pain to include physical, psychological, social, emotional, and spiritual components (Clark 1999). Our approach is theoretically guided by Saunders's conceptualization of "total pain," but with a focus on spiritual pain and an acknowledgment that spiritual needs have to be addressed in hospice palliative care for a good death to be realized.

Saunders began her work in hospice as a social worker. On an interdisciplinary team in palliative care, it is the role of the social worker to elicit the big picture, to explore and validate the larger context in which the patient and family experience illness, death, grief, and loss. This holistic perspective also includes a strength-based assessment in which the patient's and family members' personal and collective resources are identified and maximized as their journal unfolds. It is also often the role of the social worker to normalize the emotional investment of his or her colleagues in the work, providing support and grief education as needed while encouraging self-care and the setting of healthy boundaries. Although Saunders, in the 1960s, was operating out of a distinctly Christian worldview, and though the vast majority of those served by her movement (in the UK, USA, and Canada) would be Christians, the pioneers of hospice sought from a very early period to make hospice palliative care available to the growing communities of non-Christians in Western societies. One example of the way this was accomplished is evident in the work of Sister Anne Munley, a health care researcher and Roman Catholic nun who used a typology based on William James's psychology to accommodate the various forms of religious experiences of terminally ill people in hospice care (Munley 1983). Although she sought to make hospice palliative care accessible to non-Christians, in fact all of her examples are from the Christian tradition, a limitation of the existing research (most of which deals with people who happen to be Christian) and perhaps also a reflection of the deep roots of the Christian perspective in our thinking about death and dying.

A further and more recent development within the American hospice movement has taken Munley's interest in inclusiveness one step further and sought to accommodate the now rapidly growing number of people in the West who are interested in forms of spirituality that are unmoored to any single religious tradition (Bradshaw 1996). Perhaps ironically, this broader effort to open up a space within hospice palliative care for people who espouse often dramatically divergent approaches to religion and spirituality has in fact created a quite distinctive, consensual, and yet perhaps constraining view of spirituality. Bradshaw argues that in order to adapt to the American secular and religiously plural culture, the notion of spirituality in the hospice movement "has come to mean a universal dimension of human life, shared by agnostics and atheists as well as traditional religious people" (1996, 415). Indeed, it is this understanding of spirituality that has increasingly come to dominate academic thinking in nursing and medicine generally—and not just in hospice palliative care. The clinical consensus around the definition, function, and universal nature of spirituality (Chiu et al. 2004; McBrien 2006; Paley 2009) raises issues that are given critical assessment in chapters 1 and 2 of this book.

In chapter 1, "Hospice and the Politics of Spirituality," Kathleen Garces-Foley critically examines how understandings of spirituality and religion must be interpreted in relation to each other, especially when we consider that spirituality is often implicitly framed as "good" or at least unproblematic and religion is often framed as "bad" and problematic. Such dichotomies create confusion and undermine the ability of hospices to care for patients who describe themselves using those terms. Garces-Foley uses a review of hospice literature and her own experiences as a hospice chaplain in California (1998–2002) to show how "religion" has been downgraded in favor of "spirituality." There is also the opposite danger when religion/spirituality thinking becomes polarized and those on the "spirituality" side may be excluded. In this chapter, the author argues for a greater awareness of the way the concepts of spirituality and religion are used in hospice palliative care discourse. The portion of the title "the Politics of Spirituality" calls attention to the fact that spirituality, like religion, is a culturally constructed category promoted by particular people with particular goals. The analysis offered explains why "spirituality" has largely replaced "religion," understood traditionally as the framework for addressing spiritual care of the dying in North America, especially the United States. Garces-Foley observes that in this new approach to spiritual care, the winner is clearly spirituality and the loser is religion, especially Christianity—but she maintains that hospice itself also loses a great deal as a result. If hospice staff training and clinical practice demonstrate a bias toward spirituality and against religion, that bias will seriously limit the reach of the hospice palliative care movement when many, if not the majority, of North Americans see religion and spirituality as interrelated. By the same token, the growing cohort (19–25 percent) of those who identify themselves as humanist, atheist, agnostic, or SBNR must also be engaged in terms that make sense to them. Careful listening by hospice caregivers, with openness to all approaches, is clearly required.

Anne Bruce and Kelli Stajduhar offer an assessment of how to approach spirituality in hospice palliative care nursing in chapter 2, "Spiritual Care in Nursing: Following Patients' and Families' View of a Good Death." They begin with a historical and theoretical analysis showing that spiritual care has been a core component of nursing care even before Florence Nightingale. Bruce and Stajduhar locate their discussion in the early Christian and humanistic values that have shaped nurses' understanding of spirituality and the philosophical and theoretical underpinnings of the nursing discipline. They then examine how spirituality is diversely defined in the nursing literature and the challenges of these views for providing the conditions for a good death. Questions surrounding an assumed universality of spirituality and who should provide spiritual care are also explored. While Bruce and Stajduhar find no consensus on the definition of spirituality in the nursing literature, they argue that understandings of spirituality and good death must be ultimately defined and determined by patients and their families. They acknowledge that understanding spirituality, respecting religious traditions, and recognizing the growing cohort of SBNR people and the unique perspective that each individual holds is inherently complex. In the face of this challenge, nurses, in caring for the dying, need to engage in a reflective process to scrutinize their own beliefs and assumptions and how these can influence the care they provide. They will then be better able to listen to and understand people as unique individuals and so move away from the mechanistic view from biomedicine that influences modern-day nursing practice. This reflexive process allows nurses to recognize that they ought not to make assumptions about what is meant by spirituality for any individual person. Thus, the spiritual worldview of the patient directs the response of the nurse in providing palliative care. This is consistent with the accepted practice in hospice palliative care for treating physical pain—that is, that pain is what the person experiencing it says it is. Similarly, "spirituality" is what the dying person says it is, and it is that spirituality to which the nurse must respond in providing care. This individualized approach to defining spirituality is shown to be in line with Cicely Saunders's view of spiritual care as a concern for each individual and expresses a hope that each person will be able to think as deeply as he or she can and in his or her own way as death approaches.

In chapter 3, "Religion, Spirituality, Medical Education, and Hospice Palliative Care," Paul Bramadat and Joseph Kaufert focus on the education of doctors. Unlike nursing, where engagement with spirituality and religion has been present from the beginning, in medical schools and residency programs it is just since the 1980s in North America that there has been an effort to respond in some way to spirituality and religion. In medical education and practice (especially in psychiatry and hospice palliative care), spirituality is understood to relate to an individual's pursuit of wholeness, transcendence, oneness with the universe, and well-being. The first half of the chapter outlines the way in which in the modern Western scientific rationality and secularization have provided the context for medical education—a context that is antagonistic to religion and other nonscientific worldviews. However, as the authors show, over recent decades, medical training has been challenged by major critiques from feminism, multiculturalism, alternative medicine, and the Internet. In response, medical schools and residency programs have incorporated new forms of training that address medical humanities, bioethics, and studies of the social determinants of health. The chapter concludes with three case studies involving end-of-life scenarios used in medical education and assesses the way in which the patient's spirituality was handled in each case. The authors conclude that in spite of the presence of medical humanists in medical education, the case studies reveal a "hidden curriculum" reflecting a culture of scientific pragmatism in which it is difficult to engage in serious reflection about the spiritual dimensions of human health. With this in mind, say the authors, it is important for palliative care or hospice physicians to grapple with the ways in which the institutions in which they work and the meta-narrative of medical education have influenced the care of patients.

Chapter 4, "Research and Practice: Spiritual Perspectives of a Good Death within Evidence-Based Health Care," by Shane Sinclair and Harvey Max Chochinov, reviews empirical studies of the relationship between spirituality and health care at the end of life. Within evidence-based health care, spirituality is generally considered to be a universal dimension of human health, which is individually determined and expressed through nonreligious and religious means. Spirituality, as defined by the patient, has been shown to have a positive effect on factors associated with a good death. A difficulty is that while patients desire to have their spirituality addressed during their dying process, clinicians and health care systems sometimes seem reticent to do so. Three core elements of spiritual care delivery that are identified by palliative care patients as most important include being present, recognizing the shared humanness between practitioner and patient, and incorporating aspects of the patients' spirituality into the care plan. Spiritual issues are found to be as important as biomedical needs among patients facing end of life. With this in mind, the authors devote much of their chapter to palliative care–focused empirical studies of patient spirituality, spiritual distress, and spiritual pain. A careful review of dignity, as an essential aspect of spiritual distress in a good death, is presented along with a detailed discussion of the Patient Dignity Inventory as an empirical measure for clinical enhancement of the end of life. Finally, the authors note

many studies that indicate that the health care providers' qualities (e.g., compassion, respect, and spiritual empathy) at the
bedside of palliative patients are equally or even more important than medical knowledge or skills. Interestingly, as is often
reported by hospice nurses, working with patients in palliative
care is also seen to have a positive impact on the spiritual lives
of health care professionals. The authors of this chapter find
that while the relationship between spirituality and health care
may at times seem vague, and while (as Garces-Foley's chapter
establishes) it may be problematic to juxtapose spirituality too
simplistically against religion, a convincing body of evidence
clearly attests to the significance of one or another forms of
spirituality to patients' experiences of a good death. Whatever
spiritual perspective patients embrace, spirituality appears to
enhance the possibility of a good death, while buffering factors that diminish it. While empirical evidence provides important data demonstrating the influence of spirituality in hospice
palliative care, the most compelling evidence comes from the
dying themselves, who consistently identify spirituality as vital
to their end-of-life experiences.

Chapter 5 focuses on chaplains and other hospice palliative care staff members who feel unsure as to how to relate to
patients that self-describe as SBNR, atheist-agnostic, or other
nonreligious categories. In his chapter "Hospice Chaplains,
Spirituality, and the Idea of a Good Death," Wilson Will, a
former hospital chaplain, argues that the philosophical components of chaplaincy training position chaplains to work with
spiritually diverse populations including those who are SBNR.
Support from such a clinical practitioner, firm in his or her own
beliefs, yet cosmopolitan in spiritual outlook, can assist persons
seeking to integrate a spiritual outlook into the hospice palliative care journey. Will details practical guidelines for helping
atheist-agnostic or SBNR patients to explore their own views
on human existence and the dying process within a safe and
supportive environment. These include a discussion of the ethics involved in working with members of these populations,
supportive approaches to pastoral communication (nonjudgmental listening and interpretation), spiritual screening tools
for helping to identify and talk about SBNR worldviews, and

suggestions for working with children and other family members (especially when the patient's spirituality may diverge from that of his or her family). The chapter concludes with a discussion of how chaplains can help fellow staff members to process their own thoughts about spiritual diversity among the dying and the anxieties they may feel about those whose spiritual beliefs differ from their own. Will argues that it is important that the collective outreach of the care team be consistent in its spiritual messages and aims, and here chaplains can help by offering workshops for staff members on care for SBNR atheist-agnostic patients. Will summarizes his analysis by noting that "the ideal chaplain is the spiritual equivalent of an ethnobotanist: someone familiar with the tools and taxonomies of a wide range of spiritual systems and movements, from the structured to the eclectic, who can appreciate the beliefs and practices that SBNR patients and others hold."

The majority of the chapters in this book provide scholars—who may or may not be sympathetic to the cohort the book is addressing—with opportunities to use their ethnographic, philosophical, or empirical evidence to develop and advance theories about the many issues associated with the role of "spirituality" within modern hospice palliative care. In the final section, we offer two personal views about end-of-life care by authors who hold atheist and nontraditional views of spirituality. Patrick Grant, in chapter 6, offers his atheist understanding of life and death and of how hospice professionals might care for someone like him at the end. Grant writes that "none of us is ever quite as we are defined, and we remain to some degree opaque to ourselves and to one another." In caring for each other while dying, as in life, something escapes—and the absence, paradoxically, is our best opportunity for meeting one another authentically. Grant concludes, "The inarticulate in itself summons a recognition at once tragic and compassionate, beyond the consolations that can be given a voice. Yet neither does such recognition dispense with the voice that, taken to its limit, acknowledges the deeper human claim that always escapes it, and which, once recognized, can then also inform what might be spoken." In a similar vein, Elizabeth Causton's "Spirituality Unhinged" offers a passionate description of the author's transition from her early life as Lutheran to her adoption of a more open-ended form of spiritualty. Causton, a hospice social worker and counselor, seeks to move beyond all categories, including "spiritual but not religious," and shares her hope at the time of death for a fellow "explorer" to be there with her to hold her hand and listen to her, rather than a professional "detective" who, through questions weighted down with assumptions, is trying to classify her approach to death.

These chapters can be read singly or in the order proposed so as to gain a better understanding of how to approach "spirituality" in the provision of hospice palliative care. One of the frustrations shared by so many of the contributors to this book is the fact that while the nursing and medical literatures have been exploring spirituality for roughly two decades now, critical interdisciplinary assessment of this emerging concept and its applications is still in its infancy. Regardless of the approach readers take to the book, it is our hope that it will stimulate among clinicians, scholars, policy makers, and present and future hospice patients a greater interest in the complex and dynamic ways spirituality has emerged in hospice palliative care as an umbrella concept, an alternative to tradition, and an alternative tradition in itself.

REFERENCES

Bradshaw, A. 1996. The spiritual dimension of hospice: The secularization of an ideal. *Social Science & Medicine* 43: 409–19.

Casanova, J. 1994. *Public religion in the modern world*. Chicago: University of Chicago Press.

Clark, D. 1999. "Total pain," disciplinary power, and the body in the work of Cicely Saunders, 1958–1967. *Social Science & Medicine* 49: 727–36.

Chiu, L., J. D. Emblen, L. Van Hofwegen, R. Sawatzky, and H. Meyerhoff. 2004. An integrative review of the concept of spirituality in the health sciences. *Journal of Nursing Research* 26(4): 405–28.

Coward, H., and K. I. Stajduhar, eds. 2012. *Religious understandings of a good death in hospice palliative care.* Albany: State University of New York Press.

Kearney, M., and B. Mount. 2000. Spiritual care of the dying patient. In *Handbook of psychiatry in palliative medicine*, ed. H. M. Chochinov and W. Breitbart. New York: Oxford University Press, 357–73.

McBrien, B.. 2006. A concept analysis of spirituality. *British Journal of Nursing* 15(1): 42–45.

Munley, A. 1983. *The hospice alternative: A new context for death and dying.* New York: Basic Books.

Paley, J. 2009. Religion and the secularization of health care. *Journal of Clinical Nursing* 18: 1963–74.

Pesut, B., M. Fowler, E. J. Taylor, S. Reimer-Kirkham, and R. Sawatzky. 2008. Conceptualising spirituality and religion for health care. *Journal of Clinical Nursing* 17: 2803–10.

Saunders, C. 1981. Foreword. In *Hospice: Complete care for the terminally ill*, ed. J. M. Zimmerman. Baltimore: Urban & Schwarzenberg, ix–x.

———. 1988. Spiritual pain. *Journal of Palliative Care* 4(3): 29–32. (Reprinted from *Cicely Saunders: Selected Writings 1958–2004*, ed. C. Saunders [Oxford: Oxford University Press, 2006, 217–21].)

———, ed. 2006. *Cicely Saunders: Selected writings 1958–2004.* Oxford: Oxford University Press.

CHAPTER 1

Hospice and the
Politics of Spirituality

KATHLEEN GARCES-FOLEY

AN EARLIER VERSION of this chapter was published in 2006 when I was asked to write about the hospice movement for a special edition of *Omega: The Journal of Death and Dying*.[1] The original piece reflected my concern with the way "religion" was alternatively demonized and dismissed in favor of "spirituality" within the hospice literature and in my own experience first as a hospice chaplain and later as a volunteer from 1998–2002 in California. I wanted to understand from a historical perspective how religion had come to fare so poorly within hospice and to interrogate the assumptions that were being made about religion (bad) and spirituality (good). I was concerned that this dichotomy between religion and spirituality undermines the ability of hospices to care for patients who are committed to a religious tradition.

This volume on spiritual approaches to dying is concerned with a different group being excluded, namely, those who do not affiliate with a religious tradition. In the not too distant past in Western societies, religious commitment was normative and anything else—atheism, agnosticism, humanism, and the newly coined "spiritual but not religious"—was extremely uncommon. Hospice patients and caregivers "lacking" religious affiliation routinely found themselves visited by clergy wanting to pray for them without consideration of what they really wanted. No doubt atheists, agnostics, humanists, and the "spiritual but not religious" (hereafter SBNR) were not well served when hospice spiritual care was provided exclusively by Christian clergy. It is certainly progress that today the personal convictions and practices of patients are acknowledged and supported by hospice care workers well-versed in the language of spirituality. However, it is precisely this "language of spirituality" that concerns me because it has taken strong hold within hospice with little reflection upon the underlying assumptions associated with its use. Far too often it is assumed that the religiously unaffiliated have replaced religion with spirituality, becoming one of the SBNR. But SBNR is only one of many possible alternatives to traditional religion, and in fact "spirituality" may be a meaningless and even offensive concept to the religiously unaffiliated and religiously committed alike.

In this chapter, I argue for greater awareness of the way the concepts of spirituality and religion are used in hospice discourse. I call this chapter the "politics of spirituality" to draw attention to the fact that spirituality, like religion, is a culturally constructed category promoted by particular people with particular goals.[2] This chapter seeks to understand why spirituality has largely replaced religion as the framework for addressing spiritual care of the dying in the United States. Of course, one can find many hospices where traditional religion remains conspicuous and many hospice workers operate with great respect for traditional religion. Though the reader may disagree with me on the extent to which spirituality has "taken over" terrain once dominated by religion, there is no denying its recent appearance in hospice literature and hospice training materials. My hope is not only to shed light on how and why this new approach to spiritual care came about but to also reflect on the effects of the shift from religion, understood traditionally, to spirituality. As with any kind of politics, there are winners and losers in the contest. Within hospice today the winner is clearly spirituality and the loser is religion, Christianity in particular—but as I will show, hospice also loses a great deal as a result.

THE ECLIPSE OF RELIGION

As Bruce and Stajduhar's chapter suggests, from its earliest form as a place of respite and care for the dying, to its modern forms of in-patient facilities and home health care, hospice has been intertwined with religion. With the emergence of the modern hospice movement and its institutionalization in the 1970s, however, the religious dimension of hospice moved considerably away from its Christian roots. While it is widely agreed that hospice ought to be concerned with the spiritual needs of the dying, how to do this in a pluralistic society is far from clear. Hospice organizations describe themselves as ecumenical, nonsectarian, interfaith, and multireligious in an effort to be all-inclusive, but none of these terms has been as widely embraced by either the public or hospice workers as spirituality. Despite the fact that there is still little agreement on what the term means, in the hospice literature there is strong consensus that spirituality, rather than religion, is an integral aspect of dying well.

Indeed, a review of English-language hospice and palliative care articles and books published between 1990 and 2005 gives the impression that the role of traditional religion in hospice has been almost entirely eclipsed by spirituality. In the literature, spirituality and religion are generally defined in opposition to one another, with religion negatively associated with the external, authoritarian doctrines of Christianity and spirituality positively associated with the free search for truth, meaning, and authenticity. As has been pointed out by British scholars Ann Bradshaw (1996), Tony Walter (2002), Sophie Gilliat-Ray (2003), and Peter Draper and Wilfred McSherry (2002), the hospice literature promotes a rigid dichotomy between these terms without regard for how religion and spirituality are understood by the general public or by scholars of religion.[3]

The vitality of religion in the United States and its continued importance to a sizeable minority in other Western countries are of little concern to those who see hospice on the leading edge of a spiritual revolution. As Sandol Stodall (1991, 257) writes in her personal history of the hospice movement:

"Hospice in America today, in fact, has been part of a larger movement in which the concept of holiness is being quietly stolen out of 'church' and claimed as a quality of earth, and of people, and of all life created."

The eclipse of religion within hospice is ironic given how closely it has been tied to Christianity for two millennia. Separating the two has taken significant effort, and some residue of Christianity still remains in many hospice organizations. The turn toward spirituality is often justified as a reflection of changing societal norms. As people in the modern Western world increasingly reject religion—especially its institutional and doctrinal expressions—in favor of spirituality, hospice care needs to adapt to serve them well. However, when we consider the survey data, it becomes clear that the predicted spiritual revolution has not yet occurred in the United States or Britain (Heelas and Woodhead 2005). Even though spirituality has become part of mainstream culture, it has not supplanted religion in these countries; nor have the increasing number of SBNRs overtaken those who identify with a religious tradition. What is indisputable from the survey data is that there are a growing number of adults in Western countries who have no religious affiliation. Whether they be SBNR, atheists, agnostics, rational skeptics, humanists, or simply anti-religious institutions requires more digging. The rapidly changing cultural landscape in Western countries is far more complex than a simple shift away from traditional religion toward spirituality; rather, the landscape is moving toward more religious-spiritual diversity.

The struggle within the hospice movement to articulate and embody a thoughtful response to religious-spiritual diversity is shared by other public social service institutions in the modern Western world. How should institutions deal with this diversity? In seeking to avoid sectarianism, should they be strictly secular, or is positing a universal spirituality a better alternative? There are many legitimate reasons for social service institutions, such as hospice, to pay attention to spirituality, but to do so at the expense of religion is a trade-off in need of reconsideration. After all, it is not the concepts of spirituality and religion that win and lose in these debates, but those who find meaning in them. What has hospice lost in embracing spirituality and casting religion into the authoritarian, dogmatic role? To answer this question, I begin by tracing the development of hospice in the West and its transplantation to the United States in the 1960s at the start of the spiritual revolution. Next I review recent survey data on religious and spiritual identification and compare the British and American trends. Lastly, I explore how negative perceptions of religion have limited the reach of hospice care among those with strong religious commitments.

HOSPICE IN THE CHRISTIAN TRADITION

For almost two thousand years, Christians created and sustained the hospice tradition in the West.[4] Following the Roman practice, Christians created places of hospitality for the poor, pilgrims, and the sick. Hospices were founded and staffed by members of religious orders who believed that caring for the stranger was vital to Christian discipleship. During the crusades to the Holy Land, hospices served as way stations for soldiers as well as the indigent, sick, and dying. Before modern medicine, hospices could offer the sick little besides comforting attention and prayers, but with medical advances, many hospices began to function as hospitals serving to contain and cure sickness, while continuing to care for those who could not be cured. In her history of the hospice movement, Cathy Siebold (1992, 19) notes the decline of hospices in the seventeenth century as hospitals took over their functions. Religious orders continued to run hospices for the chronically ill or dying and the indigent who were unwelcome in hospitals. Many hospices operated in the nineteenth century by religious orders, both Roman Catholic and Protestant, and used modern medicines for pain and symptom control. These hospices can be seen as bridges between the medieval and modern hospice as they combined the traditional Christian care of the sick and poor with modern practices of skilled nursing and medical treatments (Murray 2002).

Cicely Saunders (1918–2005), the founder of the modern hospice, was introduced to the hospice concept through the Home for the Dying Poor attached to St. Luke's Hospital where she volunteered while waiting to be admitted to medical school. St. Luke's had a strong religious (Methodist) mission, but it was also directed by a medical doctor and had, since 1935, used the practice of giving regular pain medicine, which would become a hallmark of the modern hospice. Saunders documented the effectiveness of this and later, as medical director at St. Joseph's Hospice, taught the sisters there the techniques of pain medication she had learned at St. Luke's.

After many years of planning, in 1967 Saunders opened her own hospice, St. Christopher's, which became the model for the modern hospice movement. Though she borrowed a great deal from St. Luke's and St. Joseph's, St. Christopher's was unique in the degree to which it combined religious commitment with medical expertise. In comparison Saunders found St. Luke's too entrenched in the modern medical practices of the hospital to which it was attached. She found St. Joseph's lacking in medical sophistication and problematic because it cast the Christian ministry of the dying too narrowly into the hands of a Roman Catholic religious order. While not explicit in the written plan, Saunders's vision for holistic care—encompassing the physical, emotional, social, and spiritual—was a direct expression of her own dual vocation as a doctor and committed lay Christian, as noted in the introduction to this volume (see also Du Boulay 1984).

SPIRITUAL CARE AT ST. CHRISTOPHER'S HOSPICE

Although Saunders considered creating a lay Christian community, modeled after Roman Catholic or Anglican religious orders, to run St. Christopher's, she settled on the expectation that staff members would regard their work as a religious vocation. In doing so, she followed the example of Florence Nightingale, who had "secularized" the practice of nursing previously performed by religious orders (Bradshaw 1996). The Christian basis of St. Christopher's was evident from the central position of the chapel and the inclusion of daily prayers on the wards conducted by the staff. Like St. Joseph's and St. Luke's, St. Christopher's welcomed all patients regardless of their religious affiliation or lack thereof, and yet, as an evangelical Christian, Saunders was also deeply committed to the evangelical goal that every patient should "come to know the Lord." She did not want overt evangelization taking place at St. Christopher's but hoped patients would be moved to accept Christ by the loving kindness of their Christian caregivers. As the mission statement makes clear, Saunders understood all of hospice work as an expression of God's love for every person:

> St. Christopher's Hospice is a religious foundation based on the full Christian faith in God, through Christ. Its aim is to express the love of God to all who come, in every possibly way; in skilled nursing and medical care, in the use of every scientific means of relieving suffering and distress, in understanding personal sympathy, with respect for the dignity of each patient as a human being, precious to God and man. (Saunders 1986, 45; qtd. in Bradshaw 1996)

For Saunders, spiritual care was embodied in the loving manner hospice team members have with patients. With sympathy and respect, hospice workers provided spiritual care in their everyday responsibilities whether these be routine tasks or holding bedside with a dying patient (Du Boulay 1984).

At the same time, spiritual care at St. Christopher's also had the specialized meaning of pastoral care provided by a chaplain. The term "chaplain" is generally used to designate the clergyperson assigned to provide pastoral care to a group of people separate from a parish, for example, in a military unit. Given the Christian commitment of all the staff at St. Christopher's, the distinctive role of the chaplain was not always clear. Chaplain Derek Murray (2002) notes that tension often existed between the chaplain and hospice directors in the early years of the movement, but with seminary training, the chaplain presumably brought to the hospice a depth of theological education and experience in ministry that other staff did not share. Although the 1960s saw the field of pastoral care opening up to nonordained chaplains and greater interfaith cooperation between Protestant, Catholic, and Jewish chaplains, at St.

Christopher's the chaplain position was filled by an Anglican priest who was assisted by half a dozen seminary students and regular visits by a Roman Catholic priest (Du Boulay 1984).

Saunders struggled for some time over how to define the religious basis of St. Christopher's and whether it ought to be strictly Church of England or, in her words, "more interdenominational" (Clark 2002, 34). At issue was the practical need to work collaboratively with those who did not share her evangelical religiosity or even her Christian faith. Financial considerations pushed Saunders toward a more ecumenical stance, and eventually she began to speak positively of a "diversity of outlook" at St. Christopher's. According to Du Boulay (1984), Saunders became increasingly open to all faiths, but it is not clear how broadly that should be understood. As evidence, Du Boulay notes that the chapel at St. Christopher's welcomed Anglican, Roman Catholic, and Free Church forms of prayer, but this gathering would not qualify as "interfaith" by today's standards.

THE MODERN HOSPICE MOVEMENT

While Saunders founded the modern hospice movement as an ecumenical Christian ministry, the religious dimension of hospice became considerably broader as her model spread. When she spoke publicly with other health care professionals about hospice, she rarely spoke about its religious underpinnings. Her primary concern was that advances in treating pain and the concept of holistic care be accepted as legitimate by the medical community. As she explains in a letter to Reverend Bruce Reed, "I long to bring patients to know the Lord and do something towards helping many hear of Him before they die, but I also long to raise the standards of terminal care throughout the country, even where I can do nothing about the spiritual part of the work" (Clark 1998, 50).

Although much of Saunders's vision of hospice became the model for a vibrant hospice movement that was to spread within decades around the world, its Christian basis often did not translate into these new contexts. The American hospice movement embraced the model of holistic care including spiritual care without Saunders's religious underpinning. Ann Bradshaw (1996, 415) writes that with the institutionalization of hospice came "a profound ideological rejection of the traditional understanding of the spiritual dimension of care exemplified by Cicely Saunders, accompanied by a redefined concept of 'spirituality.'" To be clear, Saunders rarely used the term "spirituality" in her writings, though it has a long history within the Christian tradition (Woods 1989). As we have seen, Saunders understood the spiritual dimension of care as rooted in the relationship between "God and man." In contrast, in the United States and other English-speaking countries, spiritual care came to mean attending to the spirituality of the patient, which was understood as related to one's personal sense of meaning and authenticity (Walter 2002). To understand the rapid ascendancy of this new understanding of spirituality, we must take seriously its coming of age in the post-1960s United States.

HOSPICE IN THE AGE OF AQUARIUS

Religion scholar Wade Clark Roof (1993, 1999a) has described the spiritual awakening of the American baby boom generation in these terms:

> In their rebellion against bourgeois culture, against Vietnam, and against the political, military and religious establishments of the sixties and seventies, they discovered the Romantic tradition, the Transcendentalists, and spiritual teachings from the East that had been to varying degrees a part of American heritage but which had become stifled by an uptight, conformist culture. (1999b, 132)

Looking for a more authentic self, the boomers turned from Christianity to a growing array of religious beliefs and practices available to them, such as meditation from the Buddhist and Hindu traditions. The experimental mood of the 1960s' youth was eventually absorbed to varying degrees into the cultural mainstream where a "spiritual marketplace" developed to supply what seekers did not find in established religions (Roof 1999a). These new religious options included not only aspects of Eastern religions and the mystical traditions of the West, such as Kabbalah, Sufism, and Christian monasticism, but also pop psychology and an array of holistic therapies including massage, Reiki, acupuncture, and yoga.

While St. Christopher's appears to have been largely isolated from the cultural revolution of the 1960s and 1970s, the American hospice movement was deeply intertwined with the ethos of the times. Like many in reform movements of this period, hospice supporters sought freedom from dehumanizing and bureaucratic institutions. Those attracted to the fledgling movement were particularly influenced by humanistic psychology with its focus on self-actualization and personal growth. In her history of the hospice movement, Sandol Stoddard (1992, 231) notes the important influence of the "human potential movement" particularly on the hospices of the West Coast, "where there was much hand-holding and fine thoughts."

More than any other individual, psychiatrist Elisabeth Kübler-Ross shaped the direction of spirituality within the American hospice movement. Her best-selling book *On Death and Dying* (1969) poignantly portrays the great isolation and suffering patients experienced in a medical system that refused to recognize their terminal condition and a society that was unable or unwilling to talk openly about death. Kübler-Ross argued that patients could experience death as an opportunity for personal and spiritual growth if they have the opportunity to talk openly about their fears. She offered a psychological model of personal and spiritual growth, which stressed self-reflection, life review, and expression of feelings. In her later book, *Death: The Final Stage of Growth* (1975, 166ff.), Kübler-Ross explains, "It is our purpose as human beings to grow—to look within ourselves to find and build upon that source of peace and understanding and strength which is our inner selves." Kübler-Ross became a popular speaker and established a training center where she offered workshops on dying well to thousands of nurses, social workers, chaplains, and doctors.

Kübler-Ross's influence on American hospices can be seen in the first U.S. hospice, which was established in 1974. Hospice, Inc., as it was called, started in New Haven, Connecticut, without the public funding enjoyed by hospices in Great Britain and Canada. Hospice, Inc. followed closely St. Christopher's model of holistic care, but judging from the few references to spiritual care in the published histories of Hospice, Inc., spiritual care did not receive nearly the same attention as physical, emotional, and social care (Lack and Buckingham 1978; DuBois 1980). Hired at only 20 percent time, the Hospice, Inc. chaplain is described as part of the interdisciplinary team in some places and left out in others. In their description of the early years of Hospice, Inc., Sylvia Lack and Robert Buckingham (1978, 29) explain: "Pastoral care has always been a part of the Hospice concept; these services are ordinarily provided by the priest, minister, or rabbi in whose congregation the patient/family resides." What is most important to note about this arrangement is it presumed that patients are affiliated with a religious congregation and rely upon these institutions to provide the personnel to meet their spiritual needs. Spiritual care at Hospice, Inc. was placed under the purview of religious professionals under the direction of a Christian chaplain.

In contrast to this traditional approach to spiritual care, Hospice, Inc. staff members were introduced to Kübler -Ross's psychological model of personal and spiritual growth. Between 1974 and 1977, the only staff training related to spiritual care was an in-service on the topic of Jewish death rituals, but there were more than a dozen presentations on the psychological aspects of dying, especially Kübler-Ross's work. Volunteers were required to read three books by Kübler-Ross in addition to Collin Murray Parkes's *Bereavement: Studies of Grief in Adult Life* (1975) and to explore their own feelings about disease and dying. With its stress on the psychological aspects of dying, Hospice, Inc. pointed the way toward the "psychologizing" of spiritual care, which fit nicely with the idea of spirituality as a personal search for meaning and authenticity.

STANDARDIZING SPIRITUAL CARE
IN THE UNITED STATES

Much has been written about the loss of hospice ideals that accompanied its institutionalization in the United States (see Bradshaw 1996; James and Field 1992; McNamara, Waddell, and Colvin 1994). Here I focus specifically on how the establishment of federal funding for hospice care in 1982 and the subsequent requirement to standardize and document all aspects of care affected the way American hospices provided spiritual care. When hospice leaders secured federal funding for hospice under Medicare coverage for those over sixty-five, it was seen as a victory, but it came at a high cost. The low cap on reimbursement meant that families had to do the bulk of physical care and the hospice staff had to minimize visits and time spent with patients. Medicare followed the guidelines created by the National Hospice Organization in 1981: "Symptom control includes assessing and responding to the physical, emotional, social, and spiritual needs of the patient/family" (Siebold 1992, 122). Hospices were therefore required to meet the spiritual needs of patients, but unlike the other required aspects of hospice, no funding was allotted for spiritual care.

The Joint Commission on Accreditation of Hospitals established the standards for hospice in 1983. With regard to spiritual care, the standards are both brief and vague. The interdisciplinary team must include a "counselor" qualified to assess the patient's spiritual needs, and patients have a right to pastoral and other spiritual services. To comply with these standards, spiritual care needed to be documented in a manner that allowed transparency and follow-up assessment, and various checklists and charts were created to serve this purpose. Chaplain Derek Murray (2002, 109) describes the result aptly: "The glorious muddle of dogmatic, religious, and folk beliefs that made up the spirituality of many people is put into a defined series of statements and entered on a spiritual needs chart, and the patient is categorized on a religious/spiritual scale." Like many hospice chaplains, Murray believes that the spontaneity and sensitivity spiritual care requires is jeopardized with this routinization.

With no funding allotted for spiritual care in the Medicare hospice coverage, many hospices were forced to rely upon volunteer clergy from local congregations and, thus, follow the traditional pastoral care model. Chaplains, typically ordained Christian clergy, may be hired on a very part-time basis to coordinate the volunteer clergy. While cost effective, this practice is problematic because many patients or families are not affiliated with a religious community and do not have a connection with local clergy, due in many cases to a recent move or lengthy illness. The Medicare guidelines do not allow hospices to neglect spiritual care simply because patients or their families do not have a minister or even a religion. For these patients, spiritual care would be provided by the hospice team. Siebold (1992, 135–36) claims that this was one of the greatest ironies of the Medicare hospice guidelines:

> The hospice concept owed much to the religious men and women who found the resources and built up the political support needed to develop early programs. Often volunteer programs existed because clergy, who believed in the importance of humane care for the dying, donated their time to coordinate the programs. Not only did the regulations deny funding for pastoral care, they specified that nurses, volunteers, or other team members could provide spiritual supports [sic].

At St. Christopher's spiritual care was understood as integral to all the staff-patient interactions, because the mission of the hospice was to express God's love, but few American hospices have an explicit religious mission. Whereas Saunders could assure her staff members were mature Christians able and willing to talk about spiritual matters and pray with patients, how could nonsectarian American hospices ensure that their nurses, doctors, social workers, and home health aides were able and willing to provide spiritual care?

In the first decade after Medicare hospice funding began, most American hospices paid little attention to the challenge of providing spiritual care to religiously unaffiliated patients. According to Siebold (1992, 156), 40 percent of hospices were noncompliant or only partially compliant with the Medicare standards for spiritual care in the 1980s. Siebold identifies several problems with the delivery of spiritual care in this period: caregivers avoided providing it, nurses were unable to distinguish spiritual distress from emotional distress, and there was very little written on the subject in the hospice literature. These problems have since been addressed by a marked increase in the number of books and articles addressing spiritual care, many of which were written by and for nurses.

SPIRITUAL CARE IN THE NONSECTARIAN HOSPICE

It is important to ask what spiritual care looks like for those outside religious traditions. The solution embraced in the United States and other English-speaking countries was to align spiritual care with the new understanding of spirituality emerging in the 1960s and described earlier. The most common justification for this shift toward spirituality has been some version of the claim: spirituality is a universal aspect of human life that is more meaningful and conducive to personal growth than religion.

Persuaded by this claim, hospice manuals and scholarly articles generally distinguish between spiritual needs and religious needs. While only people who are religious have religious needs, spiritual needs are assumed to be universal. Shirley Ann Smith explains the difference between the two terms: "Whereas religion deals with practices and rituals, the spiritual part of human life refers to the inner self and its relationship to the universe and a higher power" (2000, 97). It should be noted that while Smith uses the term "higher power," in much of the hospice literature spirituality is simply defined as the individual's search for meaning and authenticity (Burkhart and Solari-Twadell 2001). All patients are understood to have spiritual needs for belonging, meaning, connection, and love, but only some patients have religious needs for such things as prayer, scripture reading, sacraments, holy objects, clergy visits, and planning a funeral ritual. Moreover, spirituality offers an opportunity to discover what is personally meaningful while religion offers narrow dogmatism and ritualism. This is why religion is declining and spirituality is growing. At least that is what much of the hospice literature assumes. If this assumption is correct, then hospice patients should have no problem with the promotion of spirituality in hospice care, but is it really the case that religion is declining and spirituality is growing?

MEASURING RELIGION AND SPIRITUALITY IN GREAT BRITAIN AND THE UNITED STATES

In recent decades, Great Britain has experienced a drastic decline in attendance at Christian churches. As sociologist Grace Davie (1996) has documented, Britons may continue to believe in such things as God and life after death, but they are no longer interested in belonging to churches. In 2000 some 73 percent of Britons identified as Christians, but only 12 percent reported attending services weekly (Brierley 2000, 172). More recent survey data reveals that belief in God has declined from 64 percent in 1991 to 48 percent in 2008, and only 56 percent of Britons now identify with a religion (Park et al. 2010). While there are still signs of "cultural Christianity," particularly in relation to major life passages, the shift away from institutional religion is unmistakable (Lambert 1999). In their book, *The Spiritual Revolution: Why Religion Is Giving Way to Spirituality* (2005), British sociologists Paul Heelas and Linda Woodhead argue that spirituality—which they identify with a "spiritual practices holistic milieu" including yoga, health food consumption, meditation, and hospice—is taking the place of religion in Great Britain. Focusing on residents in the northwest region of England, Heelas and Woodhead found that only 1.6 percent is actively involved in spirituality. Though this figure is much smaller than the 12 percent of Britons who attend church weekly, Heelas and Woodhead predict a spiritual revolution is coming to Great Britain and the United States.

The situation in the United States is quite different from Great Britain. Since the 1960s, there has been no significant change in the number of Americans who believe in God (94 percent) or who report attending weekly religious services (30 percent) (Wuthnow 2003). In other respects, however, religiosity in the United States has changed drastically in the past thirty years. At the individual level, there has been a striking increase (as high as 30 percent) in the number of those who describe God as a force or spirit (Roof 1999a), and those who claim to have "no religious preference" has more than doubled since 1990 to 14 percent of the population in 2001 and 15 percent in 2008. These shifts have diminished the number of Americans who identify as Christian to 76 percent (ARIS 2001, 2008). Among young adults, the trend away from institutional religion is even more pronounced, with 25 percent of eighteen- to thirty-year-olds claiming no religion (U.S. Landscape Survey 2008).

Perhaps the most important contrast with Great Britain is the way religious institutions in the United States have responded to the appeal of spirituality. At an institutional level, many of the long-established Christian denominations in the United States are in serious decline as membership drops, but newer religious forms, especially evangelical ministries, are thriving. The continued vitality of religious institutions in the United States has surprised many who expected religion to dwindle there as it has in most European countries. Many reasons have been given for U.S. "exceptionalism," but here I want to focus on how American churches have adapted to spiritual seeking by creating new institutional forms and worship styles. Scholar of religion Don Miller (1997) calls these the "new paradigm churches," which are often independent of the established denominations. New paradigm churches distance themselves from the traditional church model, disparagingly called "Churchianity," by meeting in homes, commercial spaces, and even pubs for an informal atmosphere of celebration. They are characterized by conservative bible teaching, contemporary worship styles that emphasize experiential participation, and small groups designed to encourage reflection and bonding. The small-group movement, which has now been embraced by evangelical churches across the country, has been an especially effective way to embrace the seeker mentality by encouraging questioning and searching for personal truths. As Roof (1999b, 134) explains, "small groups accommodate a therapeutic culture and allow for new styles of evangelical spirituality more sensitive to mind, body, and spirit." Not surprisingly, mainline Protestant, Roman Catholic, and Jewish congregations are creating their own versions of the small-group movement as well as incorporating "spiritual practices" like yoga, meditation, and dance. To varying degrees, American religious institutions across faith traditions have accommodated the desire of many Americans for a more "spiritual" religious life. New religious forms have been successful in the United States precisely because they are able to integrate spirituality (understood as a personal search for meaning and authenticity) with traditional religious beliefs. In other words, they are able to convince spiritual seekers that their authentic self and who God wants them to be are one and the same rather than in opposition. This strategy explains the wild success of Rick Warren's book *The Purpose Driven Life* (2002), which has sold more than thirty-five million copies to church-adverse seekers as well as churchgoers.

If religious communities can integrate spirituality within their cultures, are religion and spirituality really in opposition to one another? Heelas and Woodhead insist they are and that American congregations are not embracing "subjective-life spirituality" in any real sense: "Even when the language of 'spirituality' and 'spiritual growth' is adopted, it is used to speak of a life in which the individual listens and conforms to God-given rules and roles rather than to his or her inner feelings, convictions, instincts, and judgments" (2005, 61). Heelas and Woodhead conclude that religious institutions cannot foster spirituality, but there is compelling evidence that the majority of Americans have no problem combining spiritual seeking with traditional religion.

In the past twenty years, a number of surveys have tried to measure the degree to which Americans identify with religion and spirituality and what they mean by these terms. Some surveys, such as the Gallop in 1999, require respondents to choose to identify with either religion or spirituality, but other surveys have given the option of choosing both religion and spirituality. In a 1991 study of 2,012 Protestants in four states, Penny Long Marler and C. Kirk Hadaway (2002) found that 64 percent of respondents identified as both religious and spiritual. Brian

Zinnbauer et al. (1997) found in a sample of 348 respondents from Pennsylvania and Ohio that 74 percent viewed spirituality and religion as conceptually distinguished but integrated, and Roof (1999a) found that 59 percent of the 409 baby boomers surveyed identified as both religious and spiritual. As Zinnbauer et al. (1997, 563) conclude, "Theorizing about the terms as incompatible opposites and rejecting conventional or traditional expression of worship runs counter to the experience of most believers who appear to integrate both into their lives." Rather than a trend toward SBNR, these studies suggest a clear preference among Americans for integrating religion and spirituality. At the same time, there is also a growing minority of Americans who are neither religious nor spiritual—what Roof calls "secularists" (1999a). Clearly more large-scale surveys are needed to help us gain a better understanding of the rapidly changing religious-spiritual-secular landscape. There is also a sizable minority of Americans who see religion and spirituality as incompatible and prefer the latter (i.e., SBNR). Zinnbauer et al. (1997) report that 19 percent of respondents agreed with the statement "I am Spiritual but not Religious." Roof's (1999a) survey of baby boomers identifies 14 percent as "highly active" spiritual seekers with no religious identity. Particularly interesting for our focus on hospice is Zinnbauer et al.'s (1997) finding that among mental health workers 44 percent claimed to be "spiritual not religious." Though no large-scale study of hospice staff has been done, it may be that they, like the mental health workers in Zinnbauer's study, are much more likely to be SBNR than the general American public (Walter 2002).

Conspicuously missing from the hospice literature is any recognition of the fact that the meanings attributed to religion and spirituality vary widely. There is no awareness of how spirituality has been promoted by particular people with particular goals, the most obvious of which is, as sociologist Tony Walter (2002, 136) points out, "to move beyond, or distance themselves from, institutional religion." In much of the hospice literature, the spirituality versus religion dichotomy is presented as a timeless truth rather than a particular viewpoint. This often implicit assumption was made explicit in an editorial published in the *Journal of Advanced Nursing*:

It [spirituality] is not a mere cultural choice that we can take up or discard according to personal preference. It is not a plaything of language that can be deconstructed out of existence. It is there in everybody, including both religious people and those who think religion is nonsense. (Hay 2002, 7; qtd. in Swinton and Narayanasamy 2002)

Presented as an ahistorical and acultural fact, the spirituality-religion dichotomy has taken on the power of an ideology for many within hospice. Promoting spirituality at the expense of religion has become the "new orthodoxy" in hospice according to nurse-scholar Ann Bradshaw (1996).

PSYCHOLOGIZING SPIRITUAL CARE

While a handful of American hospices have a religious affiliation, such as Southwest Christian Hospice and Zen Buddhist Hospice, the vast majority is nonsectarian and accordingly claims to provide spiritual care for all patients without bias (Moore 1998). Whether or not there is a paid chaplain on staff, all hospice staff are trained to provide spiritual care as needed. In her hospice guide, Shirley Smith (2000) suggests a number of questions to help staff get a "spiritual" conversation started: "What is especially meaningful or frightening to you now?" and "Are there unresolved issues such as resentment, guilt, anger, or bitterness you wish to discuss with someone?" Once spiritual needs have been assessed, Smith (2000) offers the following therapeutic techniques hospice staff can use: listening to stories or life reviews; allowing expressions of anger, guilt, hurt, and fear; encouraging appropriate joy and humor; and assisting the patient in reframing goals so that they are attainable and meaningful.

Longtime hospice advocate and researcher Robert Kastenbaum (1999, 268) is critical of this therapeutic approach to spiritual care: "The standard operating procedures include encouraging 'talking about it,' reviewing and mending significant relationships, and 'accepting' both one's self and death."

Rather than traditional religious concerns for one's relationship with God or the "sacred" and preparing for the after-life journey, the goal of spiritual care in the contemporary hospice is to relieve spiritual distress and promote personal growth. As Walter (1996, 2002) astutely points out, there is little reason to refer to this kind of care as "spiritual." Nursing scholars Draper and McSherry (2002) likewise argue that since spiritual care in the contemporary hospice is really addressing existential issues of meaning and loss, there is no need to superimpose the vocabulary of spirituality. Walter attributes the therapeutic focus of spiritual care to the influence of Austrian psychiatrist Viktor Frankl whose book *Man's Search for Meaning* (1963) deeply affected Cicely Saunders.

In many hospices, spiritual care is not only a matter of "presence" and encouraging life review; it also includes offering patients and their loved ones spiritual "practices" such as prayer, meditation, massage, and relaxation techniques (Smith 2000). In some hospices patients are even offered aromatherapy, acupressure, hypnotherapy, and music therapy focused on harmonizing vibrational energy. Wasner et al. (2005, 100) suggest hospice staff should be trained in the use of "nondenominational spiritual practices such as contemplation and meditation." These practices are offered to all patients regardless of their religious heritage (if any) as universal spiritual practices. No mention of the historical roots of these practices in Buddhism, Hinduism, or New Age religions is made (Garces-Foley 2003; Walter 1996). This kind of appropriation of religious practices from "other" cultures—in this case non-Christian religions—is not unique to hospice care. As ritual studies scholar Ronald Grimes (1999, 150) points out, there is little awareness of the ways the idea of spirituality "underwrites the expropriation of other people's beliefs, stories and practices." The Western religious traditions of Christianity and Judaism are often marginalized and devalued, while New Age and Buddhist practices, among others, are extolled as spiritual. In the final section, I consider the implications of the spirituality-religion dichotomy for the reach of hospice care.

COUNTING THE LOSSES

Casting spirituality as a preferable alternative to religion is not merely a question of semantics. At stake is the ability of hospice to care effectively for patients and their families. Despite the claim that hospice attends to each individual's needs, the imposition of this understanding of spirituality can be, as Peter Draper and Wilfred McSherry (2002, 1) argue, profoundly paternalistic: "There is a danger that the blanket application of an undifferentiated, 'one-size-fits-all' concept of spirituality will be equally disrespectful to the views of those who subscribe to a broadly religious worldview, as to those who adopt a secular orientation." The religious commitments of patients are ignored in this model, and those with interest in neither religion nor spirituality are provided with spiritual care, often without their knowledge or consent. In these instances, attention to spirituality ceases to be a means of inclusion and support and becomes a mechanism for exclusion and neglect of patient and family needs (Gilliat-Ray 2003).

Could the promotion of spirituality and devaluing of religion be responsible for the lack of acceptance of hospice care among ethnoracial and religious minorities? Though no studies have been published addressing this possibility, I am not the first to suggest it. In the United States, ethnoracial minorities represent only 5 to 7 percent of the hospice patient population compared to 30.9 percent of the general public (Reese et al. 1999, U.S. Census 2000). Dona Reese et al. (1999) identify the lack of understanding and respect for African American religiosity as a major barrier to their participation in hospice care. African Americans are considered the most religious ethnoracial group in the United States with only 11 percent claiming no religious affiliation compared to 16 percent of non-Hispanic Whites (ARIS 2008). According to Reese et al. (1999), African Americans often seek health care advice from their pastors and have a strong belief in the omnipotence of God and the possibility of miraculous recovery. According to Chaplain Derek Murray (2002), such a patient would be deemed "in denial" by many hospice workers. Murray (2002) describes how hospice patients who believe in God's power to cure them are perceived by many hospice staff as "problem" patients because they are "in denial." Believing in the power of miracles and relying on the prayers of their pastor and congregation, such patients may have little interest in life review or reaching a stage of acceptance.

Ironically, in some hospice literature, there is a greater respect for non-Christian religions—such as Islam, Buddhism, and Hinduism—than Christianity (Walter 1996, Gilliat-Ray 2003). Likewise, patients who identify with a non-Christian religion may be treated differently than those of a Christian heritage. Rather than encourage expression of feelings, life review, and acceptance of the dying process, a local clergyperson is brought in to provide the necessary religious rituals. Behind this practice may be a number of disturbing assumptions that need to be considered further. Is the religious "other" treated differently because the hospice staff is only capable of providing spiritual care for Christian or post-Christian patients? Why is the religious "other" not offered the opportunity for spiritual growth through an inner search for meaning and authenticity? Gilliat-Ray (2003, 340) explains the situation as follows: "There is an assumption that 'spirituality' is for Christians or the general population at large, whatever their belief or lack of it, while 'religion' of a committed and orthodox kind defines the so-called 'spiritual needs' of religious minority groups." The result is a kind of dual-track spiritual care in which Muslims, Hindus, Jews, Sikhs, and so on are turned over to local clergy for spiritual care while everyone else's spiritual needs are the responsibility of the hospice team.

This dual-track spiritual care in hospice is troubling for a number of reasons. First, it continues a long-standing Western practice of romanticizing "other" religions as more authentic and spiritually rich than Christianity. Second, it rests on the assumption that members of these "other" religions are orthodox in belief and practice unlike Christians who are expected to have an individualized and "eclectic" approach to religion. These assumptions can only be upheld as long as "other" religions are not taken seriously as living religious communities. There are growing populations of Hindus, Muslims, and Sikhs in the United States, Canada, and Britain, but like African American and Latino Christians in the United States they are underserved by hospice. Cultural competency training for all hospice staff is a good start to understanding the Eurocentric assumptions within hospice care, but much more attention is needed to identify and eliminate religious biases, particularly the tendency to devalue Christianity while both romanticizing and homogenizing "other" religions. Until there is a greater respect for the complexity and vitality of all religious traditions, many who could benefit greatly from hospice may not welcome its services.

By failing to appreciate the continuing significance of religion in the modern world, hospices may also lose valuable opportunities to partner with religious congregations. In the United States, religious congregations are increasingly recognized as the last reliable source of social capital (Putnam 2000). Hospices would benefit greatly from better relations with local churches, temples, mosques, gurdwaras, and so forth, who can offer volunteers, pastoral visits, and financial support. This connection would also help to increase the visibility and acceptance of hospice care. Surveys repeatedly show strong support for the concept of hospice in the general public but low rates of utilization. Since clergy play an important role in their committed member's health care decisions, closer relations with religious leaders would be a strategic step toward gaining trust within underserved communities.

If hospice promotes spirituality as good and religion as bad, any gestures of collaboration with religious institutions will be disingenuous. Without serious reflection on the roots of the implicit bias against religion, in general, and Christianity, in particular, the current ideology of spirituality will continue to limit the reach of the hospice movement. This is not to say that spirituality or those who identify as SBNR should be ignored; far from it. Spirituality in all its various meanings is of great importance to a growing number of patients and their families. What needs to be reconsidered is the usefulness of opposing spirituality and religion when many people see them as inter-related and the wisdom of promoting spirituality at the risk of alienating so many who take religion seriously.

NOTES

1. Kathleen Garces-Foley, "Hospice and the politics of spiri-tuality," *Omega: Journal of Death and Dying* 53(1-2): 117–36. © Baywood Publishing Co., Inc., 2006. Used with permission.
2. Ronald Grimes (1999, 150) uses this phrase in reference to the way the idea of spirituality is used by non-Natives to exploit native religions.
3. One exception is Swinton and Narayanasamy (2002), who cite the work of religion scholars Rudolph Otto (1950 [1917]), William James (1983 [1902]), Alister Hardy (1987 [1979]), and Ninian Smart (1996) in support of the "uni-versality and enduring nature of spirituality."
4. The practice of caring for the sick and dying in special homes precedes Christianity and can be found in many cul-tures, but here I am concerned with the roots of hospice in the West, where the term "hospice" is derived from the Latin root *hospe*, meaning hospitality.

REFERENCES

American Religious Identification Survey (ARIS). 2001. New York: The Graduate Center of the City University of New York, http://www.gc.cuny.edu/.

American Religious Identification Survey (ARIS). 2008. Hart-ford: Trinity College. http://www.americanreligionsurvey-aris.org/.

Bradshaw, A. 1996. The spiritual dimension of hospice: The secularization of an ideal. *Social Science & Medicine* 43(3): 409–19.

Brierley, P. 2000. *The tide is running out: What the English church attendance survey reveals*. London: Christian Research.

Burkhart, L., and A. Solari-Twadell. 2001. Spirituality and religiousness: Differentiating the diagnoses through a review of the nursing literature. *Nursing Diagnosis* 12(2): 45–54.

Clark, D. 1998. Originating a movement: Cicely Saunders and the development of St. Christopher's Hospice, 1957–1967. *Mortality* 3(1): 43–63.

———, ed. 2002. *Cicely Saunders, founder of the hospice movement: Selected letters 1959–1999.* Oxford: Oxford University Press.

Davie, G. 1996. *Religion in Britain since 1945.* Oxford: Blackwell.

Dobihal, E. 1974. Talk or terminal care? *Connecticut Medicine* 38: 365.

Draper, P., and W. McSherry. 2002. A critical view of spirituality and spiritual assessment. *Journal of Advanced Nursing* 39(1): 1–2.

DuBois, P. 1980. *The hospice way of death.* New York: Human Sciences Press.

Du Boulay, S. 1984. *Cicely Saunders: Founder of the modern hospice movement.* New York: Amaryllis Press.

Frankl, V. 1963. *Man's search for meaning.* New York: Washington Square Press.

Garces-Foley, K. 2003. Buddhism, hospice, and the American way of dying. *Review of Religious Research* 44(4) (June): 341–53.

Gilliat-Ray, S. 2003. Nursing, professionalism, and spirituality. *Journal of Contemporary Religion* 18(3): 335–49.

Grimes, R. 1999. Contribution to "Forum on American Spirituality," *Journal of Religion and American Culture* (Summer): 145–52.

Hardy, A. 1987 [1979]. *The spiritual nature of man.* Oxford: Oxford University Press.

Hay, D. 2002. The spirituality of adults in Britain: Recent research. *Scottish Journal of Health Care Chaplaincy* 5(1): 4–10.

Heelas, P., and L. Woodhead. 2005. *The spiritual revolution: Why religion is giving way to spirituality.* Oxford: Blackwell Publishing.

James, N., and D. Field. 1992. The routinization of hospice:

Charisma and bureaucratization. *Social Science & Medicine* 34(12): 1363–75.

James, W. 1983 [1902]. *The varieties of religious experience.* London: Penguin Books.

Kastenbaum, R. 1999. The moment of death: Is hospice making a difference? In *The hospice heritage: Celebrating our future,* ed. I. Corless and Z. Foster. New York: Haworth Press, 253–70.

Kübler-Ross, E. 1969. *On death and dying.* New York: Macmillan.

———. 1975. *Death: The final stage of growth.* New York: Macmillan.

Lack, S., and R. Buckingham. 1978. *The first American hospice: Three years of home care.* New Haven, CT: Department of Public Information.

Lambert, Y. 1999. Religion in modernity as a new axial age: Secularization or new religious forms? *Sociology of Religion* 60(3): 303–33.

McGrath, P. 2003. Religiosity and the challenge of terminal illness. *Death Studies* 27: 881–99.

McNamara, B., C. Waddell, and M. Colvin. 1994. The institutionalization of the good death. *Social Science and Medicine* 39(11): 1501–08.

Marler, P., and C. Hadaway. 2002. "Being religious" or "being spiritual" in America: A zero-sum proposition? *Journal for the Scientific Study of Religion* 41(2): 289–300.

Martin, D. 2005. Secularisation and the future of Christianity. *Journal of Contemporary Religion* 20(2): 145–60.

Miller, D. E. 1997. *Reinventing American Protestantism: Christianity in the new millennium.* Berkeley: University of California Press.

Moore, A. 1998. Hospice care hijacked? *Christianity Today* (March 2): 38–41.

Murray, D. 2002. *Faith in hospices: Spiritual care and the end of life.* London: Society for Promoting Christian Knowledge.

Otto, R. 1950 [1917]. *The idea of the holy.* Translated by John W. Harvey. Oxford: Oxford University Press.

Park, A., J. Curtice, K. Thomson, M. Phillips, E. Clery, and

S. Butt, eds. 2010. *British social attitudes 2009–2010*. The 26th report. London: Sage.

Parkes, C. M. 1975. *Bereavement: Studies of grief in adult life*. Middlesex: Penguin.

Putnam, R. 2000. *Bowling alone: The collapse and revival of American community*. New York: Simon & Schuster.

Reese, D., R. E. Aher, S. Nair, J. D. O'Faire, and C. Warren. 1999. Hospice access and use by African Americans: Addressing cultural and institutional barriers through participatory action research. *Social Work* 44(6): 549–59.

Roof, W. C. 1993. *A generation of seekers: The spiritual journeys of the baby boom generation*. New York: HarperSanFrancisco.

———. 1999a. *Spiritual marketplace: Baby boomers and the remaking of American religion*. Princeton: Princeton University Press.

———. 1999b. Contribution to "Forum on American Spirituality." *Journal of Religion and American Culture* (Summer): 131–39.

Saunders, C. 1981. Foreword. In *Hospice: Complete care for the terminally ill*, ed. J. M. Zimmerman. Baltimore: Urban & Schwarzenberg, ix–x.

———. 1988. The modern hospice. In *In quest of the spiritual component of care for the terminally ill*, ed. F. Wald. New Haven, CT: Yale University School of Nursing.

———. 2006. *Cicely Saunders: Selected writings 1958–2004*. Oxford: Oxford University Press.

Siebold, C. 1992. *The hospice movement: Easing death's pains*. New York: Twayne Publishers.

Smart, N. 1996. *The religious experience of mankind*, 5th edition. New Jersey: Prentice Hall.

Smith, S. A. 2000. *Hospice concepts: A guide to palliative care in terminal illness*. Champaign, IL: Research Press.

Stodall, Sandol. 1991. *The hospice movement: A better way of caring for the dying*. New York: Vintage Books.

Swinton, J., and A. Narayanasamy. 2002. Response to a critical view of spirituality and spiritual assessment. *Journal of Advanced Nursing* 40(2): 158–60.

U.S. Census Bureau. 2000. State and County QuickFacts. Data derived from Population Estimates, 2000 Census of Population and Housing. http://quickfacts.census.gov/qfd/states/00000.html.

U.S. Landscape Survey. 2008. Pew Forum.

Wald, F. 1972. An address delivered to the Inauguration of the School of Nursing and Installation of Dean Loretta Ford, December 8–9, University of Rochester, Rochester, New York, quoted in DuBois (1980 95ff.).

———, ed. 1986. *In quest for the spiritual component of care for the terminally ill*. New Haven, CT: Yale University Press.

Walter, T. 1996. Developments in spiritual care of the dying. *Religion* 26: 353–63.

———. 2002. Spirituality in palliative care: Opportunity or burden? *Palliative Medicine* 16: 133–39.

Warren, R. 2002. *The purpose driven life*. Grand Rapids, MI: Zondervan.

Wasner, M., C. Longaker, and G. Borasio. 2005. Effects of spiritual care training for palliative care professionals. *Palliative Medicine* 19: 99–104.

Woods, R. 1989. *Christian spirituality: God's presence through the ages*. Chicago: Thomas More Press.

Wuthnow, R. 1996. *Sharing the journey: Support groups and America's new quest for a community*. London: The Free Press.

———. 2003. *All in sync: How music and art are revitalizing American religion*. Berkeley: University of California Press.

Zimmerman, J. 1986. *Hospice: Complete care for the terminally ill*, 2nd edition. Baltimore: Urban & Schwarzenberg.

Zinnbauer, B., et al. 1997. Religion and spirituality: Unfuzzying the fuzzy. *Journal for the Scientific Study of Religion* 36(4): 549–64.

CHAPTER 2

Spiritual Care in Nursing

Following Patients' and Families' View of a Good Death

ANNE BRUCE AND KELLI I. STAJDUHAR

Helen was a sixty-two-year-old woman admitted to the palliative care unit with advanced metastatic breast cancer. She never married and had a close relationship with her sister and brother-in-law; they spent holidays together traveling as a family. In the last week of her life Helen became distressed and inconsolable. She felt she had not loved or received enough love in her life. She would wake up sobbing and crying with this painful realization.

The palliative team wondered if she possibly had an organic brain syndrome but this was never confirmed. The nurses spent time holding, touching, and soothing her as best they could in that moment until she died. I know for us (nurses), we couldn't reassure her—you can't offer empty reassurances that "oh no, you were well loved and your sister loves you.'" Her reality was otherwise. All we could do was demonstrate love and compassion in the moment and hopefully that made a difference. Whether it did or not for Helen . . . we will never really know.[1]

SPIRITUAL CARE IS multifaceted with little agreement on what it looks like or how to define it. Nevertheless, assessing and meeting the spiritual needs of people who are dying and their significant others has long been considered a dimension of holistic palliative care and is a central feature of Cicely Saunders's notion of a "good death" (Puchalski 2007). Since others in this volume have explored at length the issues that surround people who define spirituality positively and in juxtaposition to religion, the purpose of this chapter is to explore spiritual care as a core and often unquestioned component of nursing care that is closely tied to the historical and theoretical roots of the profession. We locate our discussion in early Christian and humanistic values that have shaped nurses' understanding of spirituality and the philosophical and theoretical underpinnings of the nursing discipline. Next, we examine how spirituality is diversely defined in nursing literature and the challenges and implications of these views for providing the conditions for a "good death." Questions addressing an assumed universality of spirituality and who should provide spiritual care are also explored. While there is no consensus on the definition of spirituality in the nursing literature, we take the position that understandings of spirituality and a "good death" must be ultimately defined and determined by patients and their families.

HISTORICAL ROOTS OF SPIRITUALITY IN NURSING

Nursing as a profession, will embrace more than an art and a science; it will be a blending of three factors: the art and science; and the spirit of unselfish devotion to a cause primarily concerned with helping those who are physically, mentally, or spiritually ill. (Price 1954, qtd. in O'Brien 2008, 6)

Spirituality in the context of Christian service, where spirituality and religion are used to mean the same thing, has been an important aspect in nursing even before the early writings of Florence Nightingale (1820–1910). In the eighteenth and nineteenth centuries, most formal nursing care was provided by religious orders of nuns where care was an extension of devotional practice (Carson 1989). In Canada, nuns from the Hospitalières de la Miséricorde de Jesus cared for the sick in Quebec beginning in 1639. Later, in 1738, the Grey Nuns under the leadership of Marguerite d' Youville became visiting nurses (Ross Kerr 1991). Similarly, in the United States, Sister Elizabeth Seton established an American religious order that later merged with a worldwide community of Sisters of Charity founded by St. Vincent de Paul. Elizabeth Seton's extraordinary work as a nun and nurse gave her the distinction of being the first American-born person to be canonized in the Catholic Church (Carson 1989).

While these early Christian orders cared for the sick and infirm, Florence Nightingale provided the foundation for what is known today as modern nursing. It was Nightingale's use of statistics during the Crimean War and her establishment in 1860 of the first school of nursing at St. Thomas Hospital in London that laid the basis for nursing as both artistry in caring and scientific practice (Nelson and Rafferty 2010). More importantly, Nightingale's Christian beliefs provided an overarching motivation for nursing as devotional service, and she underscored the importance of spirituality as an inherent human resource for healing (Nightingale 1860; Macrae 1995).

While the emphasis on the art or science of nursing continues to be debated, there is little doubt that nursing was affected in the twentieth century both by a privileging of science and the increasing separation of church and state. Over time, hospitals and health care systems were established without being tied to religious institutions. Developmental changes in nursing as a profession in the areas of scientific inquiry, technology, and education resulted in closer alignment with a biomedical model; as a consequence, the centrality of spiritual care in nursing waned. The push to develop secular nursing science and nursing research overshadowed the art of nursing and "the spirit of unselfish devotion to a cause primarily concerned with helping those who are physically, mentally, or spiritually ill" (Price 1954, qtd. in O'Brien 2008, 6). Even so, Nelson (1995) suggests that Christian doctrine was not lost from nursing but merely transformed. She claims that Christian belief continues

to be embedded in many nursing discourses but is now identified as a form of humanism reflective of secular societies
where belief in human dignity, values, and capacities dominate:
"Humanism in nursing has resurrected the religious discourse
and the spiritual dimension of nursing" (37).

In particular, the humanistic concept of holistic care is
highly valued in nursing overall and most notably in palliative
care practice as illustrated by Saunders's notion of total pain
(see the introduction to this volume). The assumption of people
as holistic beings is a central tenet in many contemporary nursing school curricula. Beliefs underlying holistic practice include
the notion that "the mind, body, and spirit are interdependent;
the human spirit is the core of the person; a person's attitude
and beliefs toward life are major etiological factors in health
and disease" (Freeman 2003, 165). Perhaps we have come full
circle in the twenty-first century with increased interest by nurse
scholars to redefine and revisit understandings of spirituality in
relation to health and healing.

In summary, the overall unquestioned assumption of spirituality as a universal human quality can be linked to Florence
Nightingale's view of spirituality as an inherent human charac-
teristic and as a powerful resource for healing (Macrae 1995).
Spirituality is deemed essential to providing holistic care; that
is, attending to all dimensions of a person's body, mind, and
spirit (Hardin and Kaplow 2005; Smith 2006). Consequently,
assumptions of spirituality arising from Christian traditions
and the legacy of Florence Nightingale have been central to
nursing throughout its evolution as a profession and discipline.

THEORETICAL ROOTS:
NURSING AS THE ART OF CARING

In addition to the historic roots of spirituality, it is helpful for
us to describe the theoretical place of spirituality in nursing
and its implications for providing a good death. In order to
highlight the important (albeit unquestioned) role of spirituality in nursing, in this section we discuss key concepts including

caring, holism, the art of nursing, and the particular ways some theorists understand the nature of nursing. For example, caring is one of the concepts that has fuelled theoretical debates about the essence of nursing. It has been held by most nurses as one of the important features of nursing practice and by others as both the essence and central theme of nursing. A fundamental value associated with caring is the preservation of dignity, integrity, and quality of life of patients in living and dying. While caring is not unique to the nursing profession, Roach (1992) claims that it is in nursing that one sees the unique "professionalization of the human capacity to care" (41). In this way, caring is not only a sentiment but is informed nursing action and the backdrop for understanding spirituality as an integral aspect of nursing practice.

In addition to the centrality of caring as a core concept, nursing theorists have generated knowledge and research methodologies since the 1970s that support the significance of spiritual care in health and healing. Theories that fall within the category of humanistic nursing models are rooted in the human sciences rather than the natural sciences of medicine (Marriner-Tomey and Alligood 2006) and clearly exemplify holistic (mind-body-spirit) approaches to nursing practice.

Nursing as human science

Underlying the notion of a "good death" are philosophical assumptions embedded in how health professionals conceptualize what it means to be a person. To demonstrate how nursing sciences have differed from natural sciences in conceptualizing personhood, we briefly introduce the human science perspectives of two prominent nurse theorists, Jean Watson and Rosemary Parse. While their views are not reflective of all nurses or the discipline in general, they illustrate how nurse theorists have grappled with the nature of being human and the complexities of human health and illness.

From a human science perspective, people are viewed as complex, evolving beings, interconnected with the universe

(Watson 1985). The personal meanings of people's realities are considered of central importance in the investigations and practices of human science disciplines (Pilkington 2005). The concept of a person as an assemblage of traits and variables is not consistent with a human science perspective such as Watson's theory of human caring (1985, 1999, 2005) and Parse's theory of human becoming (1981, 1998, 2007). This becomes significant and is discussed further later on as we emphasize how nursing theorists have presented unique views of human health and the implications for spiritual care in nursing those at the end of life.

According to Watson (1999), the goal of nursing is to help people achieve "a higher degree of harmony within the mind, body, and soul which generates self-knowledge, self-reverence, self-healing, and self-care processes" (49). Caring, as Watson uses it, is fundamentally a spiritual act. Watson uses more overtly spiritual language while Parse's human becoming theory is rooted in existentialist philosophy and presents a different perspective. Nevertheless, the overtones of spirit and spirituality are evident and illustrate how nursing theory has been shaped in different ways by these ideas beyond natural sciences perspectives.

For Parse (2002), a person is a unitary being who through an open interchange with the universe cocreates rhythmical patterns. Human-universe is a unified concept and a nonlinear process wherein persons are continuously creating their lives in simultaneous interrelationship with the environment. Meaning making is the primary focus of choice in this perspective, and as we make choices and decisions based on our values, both limitations and opportunities are created. Human beings have the freedom to choose, which happens on many levels of awareness. We create unique patterns of living through the choices we make in our lives (Parse 1981), which lead to our unique ways of dying. The meanings we hold reflect our values and create a value structure of reality that is not limited by the linear (two-dimensional) conceptualizations of time and space. Human beings are constantly in a process of becoming as we choose among the myriad of unfolding possibilities in the universe (Parse 1998).

Nursing within this theoretical view is directed toward helping people to actualize quality of life, which includes quality of dying from the patient's perspective. A nurse's major focus when using this theoretical lens is *to be with* people as they experience their lives and eventual deaths, supporting the choosing of possibilities while focusing on the meaning the person or family gives to the situation (Parse 1992), be it life or the aims of a comfortable death. Questions such as *should nurses identify patients' spiritual or religious needs and intervene* do not arise because the aim is not primarily to intervene but to assist families in choosing possibilities within the meaning the families hold and the constraints of the clinical setting.[2]

DEFINING SPIRITUALITY FOR NURSING

I was doing night duty in an extended-care unit of a community-care facility. Mr. White, a patient in his eighties, was having trouble sleeping. He is ordinarily a quiet, cooperative man who lived most of his life in the North Country on a cattle ranch. He would frequently ring his bell without any specific request: no pain, no thirst, and he didn't want another sleeping pill. I questioned him about his needs and assured him that I was just around the corner and would hear him even if he coughed. He told me he was afraid to go to sleep in case he would die. I found a quiet time and went to his room to talk about dying. We agreed that it was inevitable and natural and universal. I knew he was Christian and probably believed there was a better place awaiting. Most people aren't anxious to get there . . . as long as they are comfortable. I also questioned his fear of getting from here to there—about the dying itself. I asked about his worries . . . did he have debts unpaid. . . . Wrongs not righted, forgivenesses not asked for or granted? We finally agreed that for him, it would be great if . . . when he were ready he could sleep one night and not know anything about not waking up. However as his nurse, I truly believed that no one should die alone. So I reassured him that I would check in on him regularly. He slept eventually and lived for several weeks longer. Lily[3]

Not only is the provision of spiritual care by nurses a long-standing dimension of holistic care as discussed, but it is mandated by some health organizations (MacLaren 2004). "Spiritual distress" is labeled as a nursing diagnosis by the North American Nursing Diagnosis Association (1992), and the International Council of Nurses' *Code of Ethics for Nurses* states that "In providing care, the nurse promotes an environment in which the human rights, values, customs and spiritual beliefs of the individual, family and community are respected" (2000, 2).

Despite the fact that nurses have been theorizing about and researching topics related to spirituality and the provision of spiritual care for over two decades, there is little agreement in the nursing literature about what is meant by the term "spirituality" or what spiritual needs and care entail (Carr 2008; Sessanna et al. 2007). The challenge of defining spirituality and what constitutes spiritual care exists, in part, because of diverse and divergent opinions about what is meant by the term, because of the subjective and personal nature of spirituality, and because religion and spirituality are sometimes used interchangeably, further compounding misunderstandings (George et al. 2000). Some scholars suggest that spirituality and spiritual care are difficult, if not impossible, to define (Harrison 1993; Ross 1994; Strang et al. 2002) because they are universal concepts that are relevant to all but interpreted in a unique manner by the individual (McSherry 1998). Even so, a number of definitions of and content analyses on spirituality and delineations of the attributes of spiritual care have been proposed (Cawley 1997; Govier 2000; Narayanasamy 2002; O'Brien 1999; Reed 1987; Sawatzky and Pesut 2005; Sessanna et al. 2007; Tanyi 2002) in an attempt to clarify the term, operationalize it, and therefore develop tools to measure it (Chiu et al. 2004). Some nurse scholars maintain that "until there is a clear definition of spirituality, health care providers will fall short of being able to formulate related nursing diagnoses and thus will fail to address spirituality as an integral part of care for patients and their families" (Sessanna et al. 2007, 252).

Three definitional trends

There are many approaches to defining spirituality in the nursing literature, and within hospice palliative care more generally (Clarke 2009; Sessanna et al. 2007; Sinclair et al. 2006), but three general trends emerge. First, spirituality has been conceptualized as a set of systems of beliefs and values that may or may not be related to religion (Tanyi 2002). In nursing practice, spirituality is sometimes used to mean the same thing as religion, as defined in terms of church attendance, church affiliation, and belief in a higher power or being along with notions of the holy, divine, and sacred (Armer and Conn 2001; Baldacchino and Draper 2001). Some research suggests that practicing nurses actually equate spirituality with religion (Narayanasamy 1993; Narayanasamy and Owens 2001). Carr (2008) and Carroll (2001), however, have found that nurses do relate to broader definitions of spirituality and spiritual care and often make delineations between these terms and religion and religious care. Nursing research has also been prone to using the terms synonymously, perhaps best demonstrated in attempts to measure spirituality by asking religiously oriented questions concerning frequency of church attendance or affiliation with a particular religious group (Armer and Conn 2001). Though the terms spirituality and religion have been used interchangeably, most scholars agree that they are not synonymous (Sinclair et al. 2006), with religion related to organized faith systems, rituals, values, practices, and beliefs about God or a higher power (Emblem 1992) and spirituality linked to meaning, purpose, individuality, and harmony (Narayanasamy 2004; O'Leary 2000). Although Stoll (1979) contends that individuals may express their spirituality through religious beliefs, values, and rituals, Tanyi (2002) argues that affiliation with religious belief systems does not mean one is or will be spiritual; she maintains that spirituality is a much broader and more expansive concept than religion.

Spirituality in the nursing literature has also been defined as a personal quest for meaning and purpose, relating to a person's inner essence and interconnectedness with self, others, nature, or God (Meraviglia 2004; Nagai-Jacobson and Burkhardt 1989). Definitions in this vein tend to be expansive, subjective in nature, and associated with a personal journey resulting in personal growth. For example, Narayanasamy (2004) offers the following definition:

> Our spirituality gives us a sense of personhood and individuality. It is the guiding force behind our unique- ness and acts as an inner source of power and energy, which makes us "tick over" as a person. Spirituality is the inner, intangible dimension that motivates us to be connected with others and our surrounding. It drives us to search for meaning and purpose, and establish posi- tive and trusting relationships with "something other" or things we value as supreme. Our spirituality sets us on a journey as part of our growth and development. It provides us with a sense of wholeness, stability, well- ness, security, hope and peace. Spirituality can be an important source of wisdom, inspiration, meaning and purpose. It comes into focus as critical junctures in our lives when we face emotional stress, physical illness or death. (1140–41)

Connection to the self, to others, and to something greater than oneself, along with purpose and meaning in life, are consid- ered to be critical attributes of spirituality (Dyson et al. 1997). Indeed, Autton (1980) claims that the need for meaning is a universal trait, essential to life itself. This is perhaps why help- ing dying people and their families "make meaning" of their situations has become a common intervention to facilitate a "good death" in hospice palliative care (Lee et al. 2004).

Finally, spirituality has also been defined as a multidi- mensional, metaphysical, or transcendent phenomenon. This includes, for example, beliefs related to transcendence, transpersonal connectedness, supernatural/nonmaterial dimen- sions, expanded consciousness, moving beyond the physical or transcending physicality, or an orientation toward "inte- grative energy" and healing (Goddard 1995; Sessanna et al. 2007). O'Brien (1999), for instance, maintains that spiritu- ality is a personal concept that is related to transcendence or nonmaterial forces of life and nature. Transcendence is seen as an essential component of spirituality leading to a process of integration and inclusion into a greater wholeness that allows liberation from suffering and an opening up to life and death experiences (Chiu 2000). Goddard (1995) refers to spirituality as "integrative energy" that is capable of producing internal harmony of the body, mind, and spirit. Other concepts related to power, energy, and force have surfaced and are related to aspects of life that motivate one's significant choices and inspirations (McSherry 1998; Sherwood 2000).

The various ways in which spirituality has been taken up and defined in the nursing literature has, to a large degree, gone unchallenged. Clarke (2009) argues that a "lack of critique" on spirituality in nursing has resulted in a bias in the literature toward broad, expansive definitions that result in spiritual care being indistinguishable from psychosocial care and that have focused on finding conceptual and theoretical unity instead of describing a spirituality that could be useful for guiding nursing practice. Of particular note is an assumption undergirding most of the nursing literature that suggests that everyone has a spiritual dimension that can be assessed, measured, and treated (Draper and McSherry 2002). In a 2002 editorial in the *Journal of Advanced Nursing*, Draper and McSherry state, "Like mother love and apple pie, the word spirituality carries with it a feeling of wholesomeness" (1). They further ask, "Who could doubt that the nursing profession's recent interest in this concept is a positive move, signalling a rejection of the mechanistic materialism that seems to characterize contemporary, technology-driven health care, and replacing it with a more inclusive and holistic emphasis?" (2002, 1). However, as some studies are beginning to show, the concept of spirituality used in health care, and in nursing, may not be universally recognized, emphasizing the need for caution when trying to apply the concept directly to diverse religious and cultural groups (McSherry et al. 2004).

CURRENT CHALLENGES

Everyone may be searching for a "good death," but terminally ill patients merely wish to have a painless,

> merciful death at the time of their own choosing. Surely
> that is not asking much. It is easy for society, the gov-
> ernment, and people to deny them this one act of mercy
> by spouting "moral," "ethical" and religious tenets by
> the dozen. They have not traveled in their shoes, and
> they do not know what dying is. In the end, all that
> these patients want is to die, peacefully, with dignity,
> and no pain. (Lee 1999)

The advent of difficult ethical issues such as physician-assisted
suicide, euthanasia, and redefining death adds to the challenges
in providing for a good death in end-of-life care. For example, complex questions about "when death occurs" and "where
death occurs" are often driven by technology and medicine's
ability to artificially sustain vital organ functioning, thereby
broadening interpretations of how death is defined. In biomedicine, the brain is the source of mind and what constitutes us
as persons. Notions of spirit, or "human becoming," are not
considered within these more mechanistic understandings of
persons. Therefore, when vital organs cease functioning and
physical and life-sustaining chemical processes end, a person is
considered dead. Or when a person's brain is vitally damaged,
as in irreversible comas, the person is also designated as dead,
or more precisely, as "brain dead" (Wijdicks, 2001). Consequently, what was previously a reasonably uncomplicated
clinical judgment about whether a patient is dead is now an
ongoing redefinition of what death means. The growing interest in spirituality adds to this complexity with diverse philosophical and cultural understandings of "person," "life," and
what constitutes death and a "good death." Within this flux
and flow, nurses bring their values, beliefs, and theoretical perspectives on what it means to be a dying person.

While there is no singular view within nursing on these
issues, we have highlighted one relevant disciplinary assumption found in nursing literature; that is, an assumption of the
universality of spirituality. As with any assumption, there are
implications for nursing and the impact on patients who are
dying and their families.

Spirituality as universal?

As mentioned, the mostly unchallenged assumption in nursing that life has a spiritual dimension (Clarke 2009) may create significant dissonance when patients hold differing perspectives. Assumptions of universality may alienate a significant number of people who either do not know if their lives have a spiritual aspect (Draper and McSherry 2002), or who may simply not think of their life in this way (McSherry and Ross, 2002). The risk of making false assumptions or imposing beliefs on patients and families during a time of vulnerability poses potential harm.

Similarly, recent discourse on spirituality in nursing has, for the most part, deliberately avoided terminology that might be construed as religious (Tanyi 2002). This may be due, in part, to the suggestion that one of the major hindrances in defining spirituality has been its relationship to religion (Dyson et al. 1997). As pointed out in the introduction to this volume, religion in the hospice palliative care and nursing literature, and indeed in public discourse, has tended to be characterized as rigid, dogmatic, and conservative, while spirituality is viewed as holistic, open, and progressive. What are the practical implications of this perhaps limited approach for patients and families for whom religious practice at the end of life is important?

In the quest to come to a unifying definition of spirituality for nursing, little consideration has been given to the fact that many people, as noted in chapter 1, do not see themselves as spiritual *or* religious but as both spiritual *and* religious (Sinclair et al. 2006). And, adding to this complexity is an increasingly large cohort of people who find meaning and purpose through nonreligious values, beliefs, and practices—a group considered spiritual but not religious.

Who should provide spiritual care?

While spirituality remains an unclear domain and is now being mandated as part of health care in some jurisdictions (MacLaren

2004), research also suggests that patients may not see nurses or physicians as the appropriate people to provide such guidance. The danger of making spirituality a phenomenon that can be "ticked" on an assessment form may potentially trivialize what many consider a potentially important component of patients' health (Puchalski 2002) and a central feature of a "good death" (Puchalski 2007).

Even for patients who may share similar spiritual or religious orientations with their care providers, some research shows that although patients do want their health professionals *to be aware* of their spiritual concerns (Hill et al. 2005), they may not necessarily wish to discuss these concerns with their medical team. Hill et al. (2005) speculate that patients fear physicians will be distracted from the medical issues and treatment concerns. Similarly, Sellers (2001) reports patients and families appreciate and see spiritual care from nurses more as a "way of being" than specific interventions. The most frequently identified descriptors of spiritual care in a study of patients' perspectives include: being treated with kindness and respect ("it's the little things"); talking and listening; prayer; connecting (being genuine, showing interest); quality temporal care (keeping the room tidy, not letting the patient suffer); mobilizing religious and spiritual resources (referrals to clergy, providing spiritual music or readings) (Taylor 2003, 580).

More research is needed, but some patients have reported that they do not want nurses to be spiritual care providers, based on the perception that nurses are not qualified and an assumption that differing beliefs between patients and nurses would be a barrier to spiritual care (Taylor 2003). Other participants in the same study saw nurses as appropriate spiritual care providers because nurses were perceived as the ones who recognize cues that would prompt a desire for spiritual care and are more likely to be present during vulnerable moments. Patients without family or particular spiritual or religious support were seen to benefit most from nurses with spiritual awareness.

Based on the call for "being" rather than specific interventions, Draper and McSherry (2002) argue against the need or use of spirituality as a separate concept in nursing care. They suggest that while nursing is a profession with "an acute sense of the existential dimensions of human life" (1), other concepts including grief, loss, joy, and anxiety adequately enable nurses to understand and support patients in need. They see no advantage in superimposing a concept that is neither collectively understood nor accepted. Further, their view of holistic care is comprehensive and already includes supporting patients who are attempting to find meaning in the changing circumstances of illness and suffering and does not require an additional umbrella of spiritual care or spirituality.

Healthy debate is essential in any discipline, and understanding the spiritual dimension of human experience seems paramount to nursing. However, as Sawatzky and Pesut (2005) argue, "we cannot afford to wait for a consensus on spirituality to grapple with the nature and practical application of spiritual nursing care" (20). What then can be recommended to help nurses who are often faced with a barrage of definitions and conceptualizations of spirituality and who may not feel competent to address such issues?

IMPLICATIONS FOR NURSING PRACTICE IN HOSPICE PALLIATIVE CARE

I believe that when we care as nurses, as human beings, we affect the spirits of other people in profound ways. Providing spiritual care is anything that touches the spirit of another. It can be keeping vigil with a family as a loved one struggles to recover. It can be crying with that same family when the client dies. It can be supporting a chronically ill individual as he struggles to redefine his worth and personal meaning in light of the illness and its demands. It can be a gentle touch coupled with soothing words that allows a worried client to sleep. Spiritual care is for everyone. (Carson 1989, vii)

For Dame Cicely Saunders, founder of the modern hospice movement, the provision of spiritual care was not optional but a crucial part of the overall hospice mandate. Acknowledging that dying people have spiritual "needs" and providing spiritual care was, in Saunders's view, key to facilitating a good death. Nurses who work with the dying and their families are often witness to patients experiencing "spiritual distress" or "spiritual pain." As most clinicians do, nurses look for solutions and "treatments" to best help those they care for. And, while the importance of spirituality and spiritual care are clearly acknowledged in the nursing literature, many studies also show that nurses do not view themselves as competent to provide spiritual care, referring, instead, to chaplains to address issues of concern to the patient (Carr 2010; Murray 2010). At the same time, nurses spend more time with patients who are dying than any other health professionals (Murray Frommelt 1991; Fakhoury 1998) and are therefore present to observe cues that are often subtle but indicative of a dying person's desire to engage in spiritually related conversations. Indeed, in our experience as nurses, some patients desire such connections for the very reason that they have come to "know" the nurse and feel comfortable in expressing their thoughts and concerns about issues of a spiritual and religious nature.

A common response to the problem of nurses who may not feel competent to address spiritual issues is to incorporate education about spirituality into the curriculum of nursing students (Pesut 2003). Others have suggested a variety of tools and guidelines to better inform practice and decision making regarding spirituality in palliative care and nursing care specifically (Chiu et al. 2004; Puchalski et al. 2009). To be sure, we need to address the marginalization of spiritually related education in nursing curricula (Carr 2010), and nurses may well require tools that will guide them to incorporate spiritual and religious care into their practice. Concurrently, though, we must also acknowledge that understanding spirituality, respecting religious traditions, and recognizing the growing cohort of spiritual but not religious people and the unique perspectives that each individual holds is inherently complex. A tendency when emphasizing the science of nursing has been to develop tools that can quickly support nursing assessments, with human experience often reduced to checking boxes on nursing assessment forms. This is a consequence of a health system built on an efficiency model. At the same time, the art of nursing acknowledges that tools such as these are only tools and should be applied in an individualized manner. It is this individualization of care of the dying person and family that we argue is at the heart of good nursing care and that will ultimately allow nurses to provide spiritual care that is respectful of all people, regardless of their belief systems.

In a survey of nurses, Grant (2004) reports the five recommended spiritual interventions by nurses. These include holding a patient's hand, listening, laughter, prayer, and being present with a patient. What interests us in this finding, and others like it, is that we consider these practices as everyday aspects of holistic nursing care. While scholarly debates about spirituality and spiritual care have yet to be settled, we believe listening, touching, reading to patients, and being present with patients have constituted nursing care since the inception of the profession. Based on our experiences, we are inclined to agree with Taylor and Ferszt's (1990) suggestion that none of these actions are intrinsically spiritual but depend on the interpretation of the person receiving the care. In other words, spirituality in each encounter is defined by the ways each person experiences it.

Doane and Varcoe (2007) maintain that being "in relation" with patients and families, or adopting a "relational inquiry" lens, guides nurses to engage in a reflexive process to scrutinize their own beliefs and assumptions and how these can influence the care that they provide. Such a lens can help nurses to better understand people as unique individuals, moving away from the mechanistic view that has been adopted by nursing from biomedicine and continues to influence modern-day nursing practice. Such an approach opens up the space to recognize that we cannot assume what is meant by spirituality for any individual person. Walter (1997) proposed a model of pastoral spiritual care whereby the spiritual worldview of the patient determines the response of the chaplain. Such a model could be proposed for nursing and in this way would guide nurses to become attuned to the particular and individual needs of the patient. As Carr (2010) says, "spiritual care might or might not include facilitating religious beliefs and practices, as it is grounded in the cared-for-person's own unique spirituality and what is sacred to him or her, religious or otherwise" (1279). This approach would be consistent with a well-known practice in hospice palliative care for treating physical pain—that is, pain is what the person experiencing it says it is. Taking an individualized approach to defining spirituality may well be the only sensible approach to take given the highly complex issues that arise at the end of life. Cicely Saunders would certainly support an approach that seeks to acknowledge the uniqueness of each individual. Though Saunders herself was a committed Christian, her development of the hospice concept was inclusive and respectful of meeting the unique needs of individuals at the end of life: "We are ourselves a community of the unlike, coming from different faiths and denominations or the absence of any commitment of this kind. What we have in common is concern for each individual . . . and our hope is that each person will think as deeply as he can in his own way" (Saunders 2006, 227).

NOTES

1. This narrative comes from interviews conducted for a study of existential suffering conducted by Anne Bruce. A portion of this quotation is quoted in A. Bruce, R. Schreiber, O. Petrovskaya, and P. Boston, "Longing for ground in a groundless world: A qualitative study of existential suffering," *BMC Nursing* 10(2011): 2. doi:10.1186/1472-6955-10-2 http://www.biomedcentral.com/1472-6955/10/2/.
2. We would like to acknowledge Coby Tschanz for her critical review and feedback on earlier versions of this chapter.
3. Lily is a retired nurse who shared this story with one of the authors.

REFERENCES

Armer, J. M., and V. S. Conn. 2001. Exploration of spirituality and health among diverse rural elderly individuals. *Journal of Gerontological Nursing* 27(6): 28–37.

Autton, N. 1980. The hospital chaplain. *Nursing* 16(1): 697–99.

Baldacchino, D., and P. Draper. 2001. Spiritual coping strategies: A review of the nursing research literature. *Journal of Advanced Nursing* 34(6): 833–41.

Baly, M., ed. 1991. *As Miss Nightingale said . . . Florence Nightingale through her sayings: A Victorian perspective.* London: Scutari Press.

Beckstrand, R. L., L. C. Calliser, and K. T. Kirchoff. 2006. Providing 'good death': Critical care nurses' suggestions for improving end-of-life care. *American Journal of Critical Care* 1(15): 38–45.

Carr, T. 2008. Mapping the processes and qualities of spiritual nursing care. *Qualitative Health Research* 18(5): 686–700.

———. 2010. Facing existential realities: Exploring barriers and challenges to spiritual nursing care. *Qualitative Health Research* 20(10): 1379–92.

Carroll, B. 2001. A phenomenological exploration of the nature of spirituality and spiritual care. *Mortality* 6(1): 81–98.

Carson, V. B. 1989. *Spiritual dimensions of nursing practice.* London: W.B. Saunders Company.

Cawley, N. 1997. An exploration of the concept of spirituality. *International Journal of Palliative Nursing* 3: 31–36.

Chiu, L. 2000. Lived experience of spirituality in Taiwanese women with breast cancer. *Western Journal of Nursing Research* 22(1): 29–53.

Chiu, L., J. D. Emblen, L. Van Hofwegen, R. Sawatzky, and H. Meyerhoff. 2004. An integrative review of the concept of spirituality in the health sciences. *Western Journal of Nursing Research* 26(4): 405–28.

Clarke, J. 2009. A critical view of how nursing has defined spirituality. *Journal of Clinical Nursing* 18(12): 1666–73.

Doane, G. H., and C. Varcoe. 2007. Relational practice and nursing obligations. *Advances in Nursing Science* 30(3): 192–205.

Draper, P., and W. McSherry. 2002. A critical view of spirituality and spiritual assessment. *Journal of Advanced Nursing* 39(1): 1–2.

Dyson, J., M. Cobb, and D. Forman. 1997. The meaning of

spirituality: A literature review. *Journal of Advanced Nursing* 26(6): 1183–88.

Ebadi, A., F. Amadhi, M. Ghanei, and A. Kazemnejad. 2009. Spirituality: A key factor in coping among Iranians chronically affected by mustard gas in the disaster of war. *Nursing and Health Sciences* 11(4): 344–50.

Emblen, J. D. 1992. Religion and spirituality defined according to current use in nursing literature. *Journal of Professional Nursing* 8(1): 41–47.

Fakhoury, W. 1998. Quality of palliative care: Why nurses are more valued than doctors. *Scandinavian Journal of Social Medicine* 26(2): 25–26.

Freeman, J. 2003. Holistic healing modalities. In *Fundamentals of nursing: The nature of nursing practice in Canada*, ed. B. Kozier, G. Erb, A. Berman, K. Burke, S. Raffin Bouchal, and S. Hirst. Toronto: Prentice Hall, 163–79.

George, L., D. B. Larson, H. G. Koenig, and M. E. McCullough. 2000. Spirituality and health: What we know, what we need to know. *Journal of Social and Clinical Psychology* 19(1): 102–16.

Goddard, N. C. 1995. "Spirituality as integrative energy": A philosophical analysis as requisite precursor to holistic nursing practice. *Journal of Advanced Nursing* 22(4): 808–15.

Govier, I. 2000. Spiritual care in nursing: A systematic approach. *Nursing Standard* 14(17): 32–36.

Grant, D. 2004. Spiritual interventions: How, when, and why nurses use them. *Holistic Nursing Practice* 18(1): 36–41.

Hardin, S. R., and R. Kaplow. 2005. *Synergy for clinical excellence: The AACN Synergy model for patient care*. Boston: Jones and Bartlett Publishers.

Harrison, J. 1993. Spirituality and nursing practice. *Journal of Clinical Nursing* 2(4): 211–17.

Hill, J., J. Paice, J. Cameron, and S. Shott. 2005. Spirituality and distress in palliative care consultation. *Journal of Palliative Medicine* 8(4): 782–88.

International Council of Nurses. 2000. *Code of ethics for nurses*. Geneva: ICN.

Johnson, R., J. S. Tilghman, L. R. Davis-Dick, and B.

Hamilton-Faison. 2006. A historical overview of spirituality in nursing. *The ABNF Journal* 17(2): 60–62.

Kobielus Thompson, P. 2010. *From dark night to gentle surrender: On the ethics and spirituality of hospice care.* Scranton: University of Scranton Press.

Lee, A. 1999. http://members.tripod.com/Amis_Lee/fallingtree/eu.html. (Accessed February 7, 2011).

Lee, V., S. R. Cohen, L. Edgar, A. M. Laizner, and A. J. Gagnon. 2004. Clarifying "meaning" in the context of cancer research: A systematic literature review. *Palliative and Supportive Care* 2(3): 291–303.

MacLaren, J. 2004. A kaleidoscope of understandings: Spiritual nursing in a multifaith society. *Journal of Advanced Nursing* 45(5): 457–62.

Macrae, J. 1995. Nightingale's spiritual philosophy and its significance for modern nursing. *Journal of Nursing Scholarship* 2(1): 8–10.

Marriner-Tomey, A., and M. R. Alligood. 2006. *Nursing theorists and their work.* St. Louis: Mosby Elsevier.

McLeod, D. L., and L. M. Wright. 2001. Conversations of spirituality: Spirituality in family systems nursing—making the case with four clinical vignettes. *Journal of Family Nursing* 7(4): 391–415.

McSherry, W. 1998. Nurses' perceptions of spirituality and spiritual care. *Nursing Standard* 13(4): 36–40.

McSherry, W., K. Cash, and L. Ross. 2004. Meaning of spirituality: Implications for nursing practice. *Journal of Advanced Nursing* 13(8): 934–41.

McSherry, W., and L. Ross. 2002. Dilemmas of spiritual assessment: Considerations for practice. *Journal of Advanced Nursing* 38(5): 479–88.

Meraviglia, M. G. 2004. The effects of spirituality on well-being of people with lung cancer. *Oncology Nursing Forum* 31(1): 89–94.

Murray, R. P. 2010. Spiritual care beliefs and practices of special care and oncology RNs at patients' end of life. *Journal of Hospice and Palliative Nursing* 12(1): 51–58.

Murray Frommelt, K. H. 1991. The effects of death education on nurses' attitudes toward caring for terminally ill persons and their families. *American Journal of Hospice and Palliative Care* 8(5): 37–43.

Nagai-Jacobson, M. G., and M. A. Burkhardt. 1989. Spirituality: Cornerstone of holistic nursing practice. *Holistic Nursing Practice* 3(3): 18–26.

Narayanasamy, A. 1993. Nurse awareness and educational preparation in meeting their patient's spiritual needs. *Nurse Education Today* 13(3): 196–201.

———. 2002. Spiritual coping mechanisms in chronically ill patients. *British Journal of Nursing* 11(22): 1461–70.

———. 2004. The puzzle of spirituality for nursing: A guide to practical assessment. *British Journal of Nursing* 13(19): 1140–44.

Narayanasamy, A., and J. Owens. 2001. A critical incident study of nurses' responses to the spiritual needs of their patients. *Journal of Advanced Nursing* 33(4): 446–55.

Nelson, S. 1995. Humanism in nursing: The emergence of the light. *Nursing Inquiry* 2(1): 36–43.

Nelson, S., and A. M. Rafferty. 2010. *Notes on Nightingale: The influence and legacy of a nursing icon.* Ithaca, NY: Cornell University Press.

Nightingale, F. 1860. *Notes on nursing: What it is and what it is not.* London: Harrison.

North American Nursing Diagnosis Association. 1992. *NANDA: Nursing diagnosis: Definitions and characteristics.* Philadelphia, PA: Wiley Blackwell.

O'Brien, M. E. 1999. *Spirituality in nursing: Standing on holy ground.* London: Jones and Bartlett.

———. 2008. *Spirituality in nursing: Standing on holy ground,* 3rd edition. Sudbury, MA: Jones and Bartlett Publishers.

O'Leary, J. 2000. The spiritual challenge in health care. *Journal of Advanced Nursing* 31(4): 988.

Paley, J. 2008. Spirituality in nursing: A reductionist approach. *Nursing Philosophy* 9(1): 3–18.

Parse, R. R. 1981. *Man-living-health: A theory of nursing.* New York: John Wiley.

———. 1987. *Nursing science: Major paradigms, theories, and critiques.* Philadelphia: W. B. Saunders.

―――. 1990. Health: A personal commitment. *Nursing Science Quarterly* 3(3): 136–40.

―――. 1992. Human becoming: Parse's theory of nursing. *Nursing Science Quarterly* 5(1): 35–42.

―――. 1994. Quality of life: Sciencing and living the art of human becoming. *Nursing Science Quarterly* 7(1): 16–21.

―――. 1998. *The human becoming school of thought: A perspective for nurses and other health professionals.* Thousand Oaks, CA: Sage.

―――. 2002. Transforming health care with a unitary view of the human. *Nursing Science Quarterly* 15(1): 46–50.

―――. (2007). The human becoming school of thought in 2050. *Nursing Science Quarterly* 20(4): 308–11.

Pesut, B. 2003. Developing spirituality in the curriculum: Worldviews, intrapersonal connectedness, interpersonal connectedness. *Nursing Education Perspectives* 24(6): 290–94.

―――. 2008. A conversation on diverse perspectives of spirituality in nursing literature. *Nursing Philosophy* 9(2): 98–109.

Pilkington, B. 2005. The concept of intentionality in human science nursing theories. *Nursing Science Quarterly* 18(2): 98–104.

Puchalski, C. M. 2002. Spirituality and end-of-life care: A time for listening and caring. *Journal of Palliative Medicine* 5(2): 289–94.

―――. 2007. Spirituality and the care of patients at the end-of-life: An essential component of care. *OMEGA* 56(1): 33–46.

Puchalski, C., B. Ferrell, R. Virani, S. Otis-Green, P. Barid, J. Bull, H. Chochinov, G. Handzo, H. Nelson-Becker, M. Prince-Paul, K. Pugliese, and D. Sulmasy. 2009. Improving the quality of spiritual care as a dimension of palliative care: The report of the consensus conference. *Journal of Palliative Medicine* 12(10): 885–904.

Reed, P. 1987. Spirituality and well-being in terminally ill hospitalized adults. *Research in Nursing & Health* 10(5): 335–44.

Roach, S. 1987. *The human act of caring: A blueprint for health professionals*. Toronto: Canadian Hospital Association.

————. 1992. The aim of philosophical inquiry in nursing: Unity or diversity of thought? In *Philosophical inquiry in nursing*, ed. J. Kikuchi and H. Simmons. Newbury Park, CA: Sage, 38–44.

Ross, L. 1994. Spiritual aspects of nursing. *Journal of Advanced Nursing* 19(3): 439–47.

Ross Kerr, J. 1991. Early nursing in Canada, 1600–1760: A legacy for the future. In *Canadian nursing: Issues and perspectives*, ed. J. Ross Kerr and J. MacPhail. Toronto: Mosby, 3–11.

Roy, C. 1997. Future of the Roy model: Challenge to redefine adaptation. *Nursing Science Quarterly* 10(1): 442–48.

Roy, C., and H. A. Andrews. 1999. *The Roy Adaptation model*, 2nd edition. Stamford, CT: Appleton & Lange.

Saunders, C. 2006. *Cicely Saunders: Selected writings 1958–2004*. Oxford: Oxford University Press.

Sawatzky, R., and B. Pesut. 2005. Attributes of spiritual care in nursing practice. *Journal of Holistic Nursing* 23(1): 19–33.

Sellers, S. C. 2001. The spiritual care meanings of adults residing in the Midwest. *Nursing Science Quarterly* 14(3): 239–48.

Sessanna, L., D. Finnell, and M. A. Jezewski. 2007. Spirituality in nursing and health-related literature. *Journal of Holistic Nursing* 25(4): 252–62.

Sherwood, G. D. 2000. The power of nurse-client encounters: Interpreting spiritual themes. *Journal of Holistic Nursing* 18(2): 159–75.

Shinbara, C., and L. Olson. 2010. Nurses grieve: Spirituality's role in coping with grief and loss. *Journal of Christian Nursing* 27(1): 32–37.

Sinclair, S., J. Pereira, and S. Raffin. 2006. A thematic review of the spirituality literature within palliative care. *Journal of Palliative Medicine* 9(2): 464–79.

Smith, A. R. 2006. Using the Synergy Model to provide spiritual nursing care in critical care settings. *Critical Care Nurse* 26(4): 41–47.

Stoll, R. I. 1979. Guidelines for spiritual assessment. *American Journal of Nursing* 79(9): 1574–77.

Strang, S., P. Strang, and B. Ternestedt. 2002. Spiritual needs as defined by Swedish nursing staff. *Journal of Clinical Nursing* 11(1): 48–57.

Tanyi, R. 2002. Towards a clarification of the meaning of spirituality. *Journal of Advanced Nursing* 39(5): 500–09.

Taylor, J. E. 2003. Nurses caring for the spirit: Patients with cancer and family caregiver expectations. *Oncology Nursing Forum* 30(4): 585–90.

Taylor, P. B., and G. G. Ferszt. 1990. Spiritual healing. *Holistic Nursing Practice* 4(4): 32–38.

Walter, T. 1997. The ideology and organization of spiritual care: Three approaches. *Palliative Medicine* 11(1): 21–30.

Watson, J. 1985. *Human science and human care*. Norwalk, CT: Appleton-Century.

———. 1988. *Human science and human care: A theory of nursing*. New York: National League for Nursing.

———. 1999. *Postmodern nursing and beyond*. Edinburgh: Churchill Livingstone.

———. 2005. *Caring science as sacred science*. Philadelphia: F. A. Davis.

Wijdicks, E. F. 2001. Diagnosis of brain death. *New England Journal of Medicine* 344(16): 1215–21.

CHAPTER 3

Religion, Spirituality, Medical Education, and Hospice Palliative Care

PAUL BRAMADAT AND JOSEPH KAUFERT

INTRODUCTION

SINCE ROUGHLY THE 1980S, medical schools and residency programs throughout North America have been seeking to respond in some way to spirituality and religion. These two phenomena are obviously more relevant within some fields of health care (especially psychiatry, hospice palliative care, and nursing) than in others (surgery, for example), though it is arguably the case that all health care personnel must grapple with these difficult questions to different degrees in their training and practice. Against this backdrop, we pose two questions: 1) Why has this interest emerged now in Western medical training? 2) What might those of us interested in hospice palliative care learn about the strengths and weaknesses of these efforts from specific case studies in which medical educators try to integrate religious or spiritual considerations into medical training?

Before we engage these two questions, we should observe that spirituality and religion are defined and distinguished in a wide variety of ways in the health care literature, and this ambiguity is reflected in medical school curricula (Buck 2006;

McBrien 2006; Pesut et al. 2008). In practice, however, spirituality is understood to relate to an individual's pursuit of wholeness, transcendence, oneness with the universe, and wellbeing, whereas religion typically denotes the institutionalized system within which these individual experiences are thought to unfold and to be regulated. As many authors in this volume demonstrate, there is a tendency within both the medical and broader cultures to juxtapose these two terms such that religion is often thought of as stifling the free development of spirituality by trapping it under dogma and tradition. While we do not ourselves necessarily accept this tidy polarized interpretation, we need to move forward according to what many educators and lay people consider to be the matter-of-fact definitions.

THE OVERARCHING STORY

Scholars and practitioners interested not just in the place of religion in hospice and palliative care, but in the place of religion in the West, often rely heavily on certain grand accounts or "meta-narratives" about broad changes occurring in Western states in the last four or five centuries. In fact, these narratives are present within many of the chapters of this book even when they are not explicitly articulated. In order to comment on the way in which religion and spirituality are managed within contemporary medical training regimes, it would be wise to foreground the grand narrative against which we usually set the return—if it is that—of religious and spiritual discourse to at least this corner of the medical world.

We use the term "narrative" in a manner that combines both the common and the academic senses of the term: as a collectively held general account of the way a situation has emerged. We do, nonetheless, wish to signal by choosing this term the contested and contrived nature of all collective accounts of large historical processes. However, even with that caveat, an assessment of the broad narrative in question may explain how it came to pass that religion and its surrogates (spirituality, magic, superstition, and lore) have come to be framed in a particular way by the medical staff who work in hospice palliative care contexts.

According to the way a great many people—and for the sake of simplicity, we will limit ourselves to people in the West—imagine the past, there was once a time where a fully secular life was inconceivable. This was the case until the last few centuries.

Scientific rationality, we are told, was responsible for the change in the fortunes of religion in the West. It is true that the assumed hegemony of religious expectations suffered as Copernicus in the sixteenth century and Galileo in the seventeenth century challenged the geocentric view of the cosmos. However, other forces were also at work in the diminishment of the overarching power of religion. Beyond the advent of a particular kind of scientific reason, there were, just to list the most obvious: the rapid spread of printing presses in the fifteenth and sixteenth centuries; the Protestant Reformation of the sixteenth century; the emergence of Cartesian scepticism in the seventeenth century; the long and bloody Wars of Religion that ended with the Treaty of Westphalia in the seventeenth century; the democratic revolutions in the eighteenth century (in France and the United States, especially); the Industrial Revolution in the eighteenth and nineteenth centuries; the Enlightenment and the rise of liberal democracies in the eighteenth century; the critiques of religion in the mid-nineteenth to mid-twentieth centuries related most often to the writings of Durkheim, Marx, Weber, Freud, and Nietzsche; and in the twentieth century, the rise of atheistic socialism and postmodernism as alternative ways of understanding human life and community. Although most of these movements and many of their leading figures assumed the veracity of, or were sometimes in sympathetic dialogue with, certain (Jewish or Christian) theological claims, each of these forces played its own role in what we now call the secularization of Western societies.[1]

Of course, the political and social processes that stretched from the Renaissance to the contemporary period and diminished the amount of *de facto* and *de jure* control religious institutions had over many Western societies reflect only one dimension of secularization. One also needs to consider the extent to which these processes were concomitant with a decrease in personal religious convictions. On this topic, there is debate—both about what was happening during the last three or four tumultuous centuries and also about what is still happening. This historical debate persists in part because only recently have we begun to conduct surveys and interviews to determine the significance of religion in the individual lives of ordinary citizens in the West.

In general, though, it would probably be fair to suggest that there has been a relatively consistent level of religious conviction and practice throughout the last few centuries. What arguably changed during the last hundred years—and is most evident now—are the following:

- the destabilization of the loyalty of individuals to a particular religious tradition or denomination; and
- the increasing popularity of the concept of "spirituality" in contrast to "religion"—especially evident in the growing and empirically recognizable cohort of people who describe themselves as "spiritual but not religious"; and, finally,
- the probably unprecedented possibility of living lives entirely outside of the orbit of any explicitly religious convictions or institutions.

While one could argue that forms of scepticism, agnosticism, and atheism have existed for centuries in the West, those approaches that emphasize the "spiritual" over the "religious" are not adopted merely by an infinitesimal number of elite Westerners (especially Canadians and western Europeans), but by an ever-increasing number of people under roughly forty years of age. Indeed, this shift is so new and widespread that scholars have yet to "thematize" it adequately; yet it is also probably in need of the most rigorous analysis.[2]

This is not the place to discuss the various trajectories of and debates about secularization (see Swatos and Olson 2000). It is sufficient to observe that many of the writers in this book (and no doubt most of its readers) generally assume the validity of a common narrative according to which our society was *once* shot through with religious practices, sensibilities, and presuppositions and *now*, especially in the West, it is no longer so. At this point, we simply do not know enough about this shift to make many definitive claims about its future effects.[3]

We can say, though, that this story about religion and society in the modern West has a great effect on the way we think about religion and health care. Far from being, on its own, a sufficient explanation for the way things are and have to be, the unidirectional secularist meta-narrative is also a means of underlining the necessity of the consensus around Western allopathic medical conventions. However, it is the hallmark of ideologies—in this case, "secularism"—to offer clear accounts of the ways history *has* unfolded and a kind of road map for the way history *should* unfold. It is in the very nature of ideologies that they are normative. In this case, a story has developed about the incommensurability of or the deep tensions between religion and science, and regardless of whether such differences are in fact irreconcilable, the story in itself has been a pillar of our universities, medical schools, and other parts of our civil society. This account of the way things have changed historically in our society (where we were once steeped in "magical thinking" and are now moving toward a relatively disenchanted, rational world) does not simply *describe* a world in which the religious and secular/scientific realms are antagonists in a zero-sum game, but in fact *creates and sustains* such a dichotomized world.

There is no doubt that this narrative of the gradual unfolding of scientific truth both captured genuine progress and also constituted a normative story that has brought humankind great benefits. Few of us would want to return to a time when medical techniques included trepanation, bloodletting, and leeching, not to mention a time when infant mortality and dental pain—things modern Western people expect to be nearly nonexistent—would have been a routine part of life. Moreover, the optimism that this positivist narrative has created among physicians and medical researchers is also a great boon to our societies; after all, it is this sense of the gradual unfolding of truth that emboldens researchers (and funding agencies) to continue the search for cures for diseases—cancer, diabetes, and HIV, for example—that until recently had been fatal.

In the wake of the well-known Flexner Report of 1910, there emerged in the United States an approach to the practice of medicine (and the training of physicians) that concentrated social power in the hands of physicians and in so doing exerted control over a number of other diagnostic and health practices and professionals. The Flexner Report was part of the professionalization of the medical sciences, but parallel forces were at work at roughly the same time as well in the development of social work as a distinct profession. As a result of the Flexner Report, American medical practice was definitively reorganized; in Canada (with a much smaller population and a greater openness to socialized medicine), the situation at the time was comparatively less fluid, though a wide variety of medical systems coexisted and the economic clout and social prestige associated with physicians had yet to approximate what we now observe. Nonetheless, in the early decades of the twentieth century, both American and Canadian societies moved toward the consolidation of the positivistic allopathic paradigm, a regime of truth and knowledge that would not be significantly challenged until the last two decades of the same century (Coburn et al. 1983).

For most members of our society, the ideology that validates this scientific meta-narrative has become thoroughly "naturalized," really the "only game in town." This is not the place for a full discussion of alternatives to this story, but it is worthwhile to reflect on why questions have arisen about the dominant account. This will prepare us to consider the extent to which medical training has evolved to respond to these questions.

THE CENTER CANNOT HOLD:
ON THE SWINGING OF THE PENDULUM

Medical students are often attracted to the profession because it offers them a secure form of prestige and affluence, but also because medicine is seen as noble, as committed to the alleviation of suffering and the improvement of public health. The tremendous success of medicine led some physicians—and, one might argue, the "system" as a whole—to adopt a patronizing posture toward patients and competing truth claims. Over the last several decades, however, the authority of the profession has been challenged from a number of angles, creating the conditions for what we might call the "perfect storm" of skepticism as to either its universal or particular value for our societies. Here we can list a number of the major critiques.

FEMINISM

First, for several decades since the 1960s, many feminists argued that conventional Western medicine played a significant role in maintaining the subservience of women through popular prescription medications such as Valium and condescending caricatures of women's illnesses (both of which, some contend, stifled women's political agency). As well, feminists have observed the many ways in which ambitious and intelligent young women were encouraged to become nurses instead of physicians until the last few decades of the twentieth century (Code 1991; Holmes and Purdy 1992; Sherwin 1992 and 2008).

SCANDALS

Second, scandals involving incompetent or unethical medical practices have also tarnished the public perceptions of the profession. Some of these scandals have involved the sexual abuse or manipulation of women (Cohen 1995),[4] though others have involved the once more common—and lingering—practice of pharmaceutical companies being allowed to exert undue influence not only over research, but over physicians and medical students through lavish gifts and conferences in exotic locales. In addition, during the last several years there have been other scandals related to the effects of incompetent pathology reports leading to the imprisonment of innocent people,[5] or a radiologist's fatal misdiagnoses of hundreds of women,[6] as well as intentionally manipulated data that led to widespread doubts over immunizations.[7] To some, these scandals are not surprising

and simply reflect the conventional humaneness of medical professionals;[8] to other members of the general public, however,
these events represented a further fall from grace.

IMPROVEMENTS IN PUBLIC HEALTH

Third, the success of Western medicine has, perhaps ironically, led to unrealistic expectations regarding disease trajectory, the extension of life expectancy and a perception of the
unlimited efficacy of Western medicine. Many people often take
for granted some of the health benefits that were the result of
rigorous medical research and political pressure (e.g., fluoridation of water supplies; the enrichment of milk and flour; mass
immunization campaigns to eradicate polio, pertussis, rubella,
and diphtheria). Thanks to these broad social improvements
brought about through the efforts of physicians and public
health workers, most people expect to (and actually do) live
longer and less painful lives than their ancestors could have
imagined. This is clearly a welcome development, though it
has meant that physicians are not as broadly revered as they
once were during the period when cures for these diseases were
emerging.

ALTERNATIVE HEALTH AND THE INTERNET

Fourth, the increased ethnic, cultural, and religious diversity of
many Western states, along with the rise of the Internet, have led
to the increased interest in alternative or complementary treatment modalities such as those based in chiropractic, Ayurvedic,
and traditional Chinese medicines, as well as more idiosyncratic
forms patients themselves construct out of the many approaches
on display on the Internet. Unfortunately, Western-trained allopathic physicians receive virtually no training in these alternative—and very often spiritually infused—treatments.

Now, however, those at the margins of medical power
(nurses, physiotherapists, chiropractors, midwives, alternative
practitioners) have a great deal more latitude. The legal restrictions on alternative medicines have been loosened significantly,
and the contemporary doctor-patient relationship now confers

an unprecedented degree of autonomy on the patient. In many cases, a more collaborative doctor-patient model can draw patients more fully into their own treatment regimens; in other cases, patients with often specious perspectives on their own bodies can eventually come to view the physician as merely a consultant, and even an obstacle to his or her health. Indeed, even definitive scientific evidence discounting the practice of homeopathy,[9] or The Lancet's formally retracted article about the connection between autism and the measles-mumps-rubella vaccination,[10] are very often not enough to dissuade people from pursuing their own course of action.

EVIDENCE-BASED ALTERNATIVES

Fifth, there has emerged in the medical literature itself some evidence that seems to call into question a strictly mechanistic model of human health. Consider evidence that does, or that appears to, support a correlation between positive public and individual health outcomes on the one hand and prayer and meditation on the other hand (Chiesa and Serretti 2010; Goldine and Gross 2010); clinical trials that seek to establish the efficacy of particular Chinese herbal treatments or Ayurvedic therapies;[11] scientific evidence that demonstrates the subtle and sometimes unpredictable interplay between "nature" and "nurture" in determining an individual's or a group's susceptibility to certain illnesses (Ptak and Petronis 2008); and clinical evidence of the effect of psychotherapy on brain function and physiology (Linden 2006; Mayo 2009; Sharpley 2010). In a medical model increasingly defining itself as "evidence-based," these cases have helped to challenge not just the sufficiency of a narrow mechanistic model but also the failure of the model to take account of alternative scientific and spiritual claims.

CHALLENGES TO INDIVIDUALISM

Sixth, while the institutions and norms of modern Western society—from our human rights codes to our privacy regulations to our approach to medical research, nursing, and social work—presuppose the absolute centrality and inviolability of the individual, in fact, a great many religious, ethnic, and national subcultures in Canada (such as most First Nations and most newcomer communities) operate according to a view of each individual as inextricably embedded in a family and a community (Solomon 1997). Some scholars (Coward and Ratanakul 1999) distinguish between the notion of the "I-self" that is the imagined central figure in Western societies, and the "we-self" that is far more common elsewhere in the world and in Canada within many minority communities. It is not the case that these minority perspectives on the self disregard or deny the individual, but rather that they tend to emphasize the intimate *relationships* between the self and one's community as more important than the abstracted notion of the individual. The distinctions between autonomy-focused bioethics and recognition of family or community oversight are increasingly recognized in teaching around informed consent and proxy decision making at the end of life (Kaufert and Putsch 1997). In *Religious Understandings of a Good Death in Hospice Palliative Care* (Coward and Stajduhar 2012), the first volume of this project, a number of chapter authors outlined the various ways in which the dominant medical structure that is still assumed in many hospice palliative care contexts could not adequately treat patients and families operating out of fundamentally different perspectives associated with non-Christian traditions. Fortunately, more and more nurses, social workers, and palliative care physicians are becoming aware of these shortcomings, and this awareness has created an opportunity for such professionals to revisit what one might call the "fetishization of autonomy" that is still an integral part of medical education and clinical practice in most Western medical systems.

Demography is destiny

Seventh, and finally, as even a brief trip to any urban center will demonstrate, profound deracializing policy changes in the late 1960s had a deep impact on Canadian demography, making our society both more ethnically and religiously diverse (Bramadat and Seljak 2005 and 2008). These changes have also impacted the demography of all health professions, since faculties of medicine and now the broader community of practitioners have become more reflective of the ethnocultural and religious diversity of Canadian society.

Many will contend that social institutions such as hospitals and hospices need to be flexible enough to address Muslims, Sikhs, Hindus, First Nations, Chinese, Jews, and people who profess no religion as well as those whose spirituality does not fit easily within any single religious tradition. Critical analysis of the historical legacy of religion in institutions such as hospitals and residential schools for Aboriginal people has also emphasized that traditional spiritual practice in end-of-life care may have to be accommodated in alternative community-centered care space (Kaufert et al. 2012). We have generally treated minority religious claims—for distinctive health treatments or culturally sensitive care at the end of life—as individual exceptions to the (implicitly natural) status quo. However, perhaps what is really needed is a deeper reconsideration of the dominant paradigm and the institutions (such as health care facilities) that have been built on this structure, and specifically of the extent to which this paradigm may exclude members of both religious minority communities and, more recently, those who would describe themselves as spiritual but not religious.[12]

Three Positive Changes

We have outlined the development of the meta-narrative that undergirds Western medical training (and indeed, Western discourse on the body, science, and technology) and seven ways that story has been assailed in recent history. Obviously, medical schools and residency programs are not static, and indeed both—though probably medical schools more than residency programs—have responded in a number of ways to these challenges. We can describe at least three of them prior to reflecting on case studies that will allow us to assess the depth and effectiveness of the responses.

MEDICAL HUMANITIES

Over the past fifteen years, some Canadian faculties of medicine have introduced blocks into the undergraduate curriculum under the heading of alternative and complementary therapies. Often, but not always, these blocks comprise initiatives in the "medical humanities" programs within these medical schools. In these modules, homeopathic, chiropractic, and naturopathic practitioners are typically asked to present an overview of their alternative philosophical foundations and scope of practice with a view to informing physicians' management of patients who use multiple alternative healing practices, some of which might be contraindicated when a patient is also using allopathic practices and medicines, some of which might be merely placebos unsupported by any scientific evidence, and some of which might be inherently dangerous.

Initially, medical traditions such as Ayurvedic and Chinese medicine, which are thousands of years old, were each covered in less than thirty minutes.[13] However, in the past decade, several faculties of medicine have offered optional clinical placements within complementary medical settings and more comprehensive overviews of Ayurvedic medicine, Islamic medical practice, traditional Chinese medicine, and traditional Aboriginal healing practices. Inclusion of these systems of knowledge and practice in the curriculum increasingly encourages students to be aware of the formal religious beliefs and practices and the less well-defined spiritual beliefs and practices that form the basis for healing practice and ethical decision making for so many people. As further evidence of this relatively recent and relatively friendly approach, we see a widespread interest in spirituality (often through "mindfulness" meditation, which is, in essence, Buddhist meditation without its religious trappings) within the palliative care community—as a consideration of the most recent international conference on palliative care (Montreal, October 2010)[14] demonstrates. At the McGill University Faculty of Medicine in Montreal, we also see a turn toward "whole person care"[15] and the growth in an ever-expanding social work, medical, and nursing literature on the spirituality and well-being of patients and medical personnel. The development over the past decade of a separate Indigenous health curriculum at the University of Manitoba, for example, has introduced teaching modules related to (and often optional participation in) sweat lodge ceremonies, as well as teaching by

Aboriginal elders that exposes medical students to traditional Cree, Ojibway, and Dene spiritual practices related to healing, death, and spiritual continuity.

BIOETHICS

As a reflection of a growing consensus within medical education and the broader society that students need to be exposed to a wider range of issues from the social sciences, moral philosophy, and other areas of the medical humanities, one can see since the popularization of the Belmont principles a growing interest in bioethics as a distinctive area of intellectual inquiry. The *Belmont Report* (National Commission for the Protection of Human Subjects 1978) defined key principles that were to form the center of evaluation of the ethical dimension of both clinical and research relationships in biomedical health services and health services research. Although this document was produced in the United States, it had effects on the development of bioethics around the world. Two effects of the Belmont principles have been recognition of pluralism in the way ethical principles such as autonomy are interpreted by minority ethnocultural or religious groups. For example, there is an awareness that while respect for individual autonomy is promoted (actually, assumed) in most medical educational settings and in clinical and research consent agreements, there is an interest, as well, in presenting some cross-cultural examples to students that recognize that some religious and ethnocultural groups place more emphasis on the rights of the family or community (especially Aboriginal and Muslim groups) as a collectivity than on the rights of the individual (Kaufert and Putsch 1997).

SOCIAL DETERMINANTS OF HEALTH

Although evidence-based medical education is still deeply rooted in the positivist tradition, it increasingly focuses on the "social determinants of health," an epidemiologically informed concept that moves beyond an interest simply in a patient's body and attempts to factor into research and practice a broader critical awareness of the health effects of the environment,

lifestyle choices, social supports, and public policy. At a population level, these models are expanded to include the influence
of religious pluralism and spirituality as sources of social capital and physical and social resilience. For example, these models—increasingly popular in medical schools and public health
units—have encouraged students to elicit information from
their patients on the dimension of spirituality. Engel's original
1978 formulation[16] of the "biopsychosocial" model has been
extended, initially in the field of gerontology, to become the
"biopsychosocial-spiritual" model.[17]

LESSONS FROM CLINICAL PRACTICE

Now that we have outlined three responses to the major critiques of a deeply embedded allopathic medical system, we can
reflect on the extent to which the medical education system
has responded to these concerns. Three case studies herein will
enable us to assess the efforts made by medical educators to provide training related to the religious and spiritual backgrounds
of their patients.[18] While these case studies are not themselves
based exclusively in palliative care settings, they speak volumes
about the educational processes involved in training physicians.

Case Study 1: Spirituality and Cultural Miscommunication

A Cree-speaking elder with advanced diabetes-related vascular
insufficiency developed a life-threatening infection in her leg
and was admitted to hospital.[19] A vascular surgeon asked her
family for permission to speak with the elder so that he might
explain her life-threatening situation and limited treatment
options. The elder only spoke Cree and needed an interpreter,
but a member of the family, who had accompanied her to hospital, said that she had worked as an interpreter at a regional
hospital and could translate for her mother. The translation by
the family member did not engage the issue of mortality risk
and high probability of need for additional "limb salvaging surgery." Following the daughter's explanation, the elder signed

the printed version of the agreement in English. The surgery to restore the blood supply to her lower leg and foot surgery went ahead and left her with a surgical wound extending from her upper thigh to her ankle.

When Cree-speaking interpreters from the hospital's Aboriginal services department visited the elder after the surgery, they found that she was profoundly depressed and very angry, complaining that neither the doctor nor her daughter had prepared her for the level of postoperative trauma. She was particularly angry with her daughter because she stated that her daughter was "a devout Christian" and had not communicated the risk of limb loss in terms of her spiritual beliefs. Two days after the initial surgery, the elder's condition deteriorated, the infection progressed, and her leg became gangrenous. The team and daughter agreed that the elder had diminished competence as she lapsed in and out of consciousness. The surgical amputation of the elder's lower leg was completed, but over the next three days, the patient experienced multiple organ failure and died with her extended family around her.

The case was initially used to emphasize the importance of cross-cultural communication and the impact of professional or family interpreters. However, the underlying issue in this case was that due to the absence of a culturally sensitive professional translator who might have been able to engage spiritual concerns and concepts in a responsible manner, the diabetic elder was unable to explain that according to her traditional spiritual beliefs, surgical amputation would compromise her corporal integrity when she "passed into the afterlife." In these sessions, the content of the patient's traditional beliefs was not engaged, and elders with knowledge of Cree language and traditions who might have elucidated these beliefs were not included in the teaching team.

Over the past five years at the University of Manitoba, the participation in the teaching sessions of an Aboriginal elder with knowledge and involvement in traditional spiritual practices has introduced into medical education a wider explanatory framework in which the patient's decision about refusing life-preserving treatment can be more fully understood in terms of her spiritual beliefs. In Manitoba, clinical observations suggested that the inclusion of the elder enabled students to understand these beliefs and consider alternatives to surgical amputation, including referral to palliative care units with capacity to engage the spiritual context of dying within a culturally appropriate "safe space" (Kaufert et al. 2011).

Professionals and other caregivers involved in hospice palliative care can learn three lessons from this case study. First, it is important to recognize and clarify the impact of alternative spiritual values and formal religious beliefs among patients and family members. Second, it is important to recognize that informal interpreters and proxy decision makers communicating the decisions of dying family members may block or modify the translation or interpretation of the patient's choices about end-of-life care. Third, it is important to involve members of the patient's religious and cultural community (outside of the family) to enable to the hospice palliative care team to interpret the individual choices and spiritual context of the person's or family's decisions at the end of life.

Case Study 2: Generic Reference to Spirituality

A woman who had immigrated to Canada five years ago from Eastern Europe was admitted to hospital with congestive heart failure and required emergency cardiac surgery during the second trimester of her pregnancy.[20] The woman was forty years old, and her clinical records indicated that she had had two previous miscarriages. The woman underwent an emergency Caesarean section in the seventh month of her pregnancy, but the baby survived only twenty-four hours.

Her cardiologists and gynecologists advised her that another pregnancy would place both her own life and the life of the fetus at risk. Eight months later, the woman consulted her family doctor, at which point he discovered that she was close to the end of her first trimester. She told her physician that she was determined to continue with the pregnancy despite the high risk of mortality for herself and the strong possibility that the infant would not survive.

The actual teaching case did not describe the outcome of the women's decisions (for herself or her fetus), but for our purposes this is not relevant. The important observation is that the possibility that the continuation of pregnancy would lead to the woman's death was not linked to religious questions. In fact, the notes for tutorial leaders encouraged students to consider the patient's "beliefs" regarding the importance of childbearing, the value of children, and her particular family dynamics. They were also asked to consider the impact of the woman's background as a recent immigrant, her medical history in Canada, and the loss of three children. Students were asked to discuss some of the following questions: What factors would you want to consider in determining why she stopped using contraception and became pregnant? Do you think she was influenced by her husband, her family, or her community? Did she fully understand the risk for herself in becoming pregnant again? Was she influenced by the loss of her other pregnancies?

These are certainly among the relevant questions physicians would want to pose. However, the questions avoid any reference to the potential impact of religion or spirituality on the patient's decision. Even though the teaching module was presented in a section of the human development curriculum that emphasized engaging (among other factors) a "spiritual dimension" through the application of the biopsychosocial-spiritual model described earlier, there seemed to be a reluctance among instructors and curriculum developers to engage students in discussions of the relationships between religion and decisions related to mortality, risk, and values. In fact, tutorial leaders were actually advised to tell students that the woman had not identified with any particular religion. This is most unfortunate, since it is at least conceivable that her spiritual or religious beliefs played some role in her judgment about the risk of death associated with her pregnancy, and yet the way this case was constructed betrays an effort to steer students away from this particular set of questions.

In this case, we can make three observations. First, while student physicians learn about mortality, risks of dying, and end-of-life decision making in many other areas of the curriculum than simply the medical humanities, such cases could provide an opportunity to address in a systematic and open manner the impact of religion and spirituality on clinical practice and patients' decisions. Second, the case appears to be designed to exclude religious and spiritual concerns altogether, even though the bare facts of the case—a forty-year-old woman from a region with which very few Canadian caregivers would have any familiarity (but in which religion has often been a "problematized" social force)—suggest there would be religious or spiritual ideas at work.

Third, this case study reflects a discomfort within medical education in general with some of the more complicated features of religion and spirituality in the contemporary West. In particular, in order to engage some of the deeper motivations for the patient's unusual health decisions, the health professionals would arguably need to consider the ways in which religious or spiritual perspectives intersect with notions of gender, nationalism, or citizenship status. The connections between religion and these additional identities are complicated and can only be evinced through meaningful and extensive communication. This case seems to be designed to prevent such discussions.

Case Study 3: Public Controversies Related to Religion, Spirituality, and Life-Supporting Treatment

Mr. Golubchuk was eighty-four years old and experienced cognitive impairment after falling and increasing disability associated with the progression of multiple chronic conditions. The patient was admitted to an intensive care unit and was supported through tube feeding and mechanical ventilation. His attending physicians assessed his cognitive status and concluded "that he was hardly able to respond to his environment." The physicians in the intensive care unit also stated that the patient was unlikely to recover and argued for a care plan that would allow them to "remove the artificial interventions and allow him to die naturally" (Pauls 2011, 1).

Mr. Golubchuk's son and daughter argued for continuation of the treatment interventions because their father could interact with the family and community in "some small way." They also stated that their Jewish faith prohibited them "from agree-ing to actions (including removing treatments) that might has-ten their father's death" (Pauls 2011, 1).

The attending physicians in the ICU of the hospital caring for Mr. Golubchuk referred to the College of Physician's policy guidelines treatment decisions involving withholding or with-drawing care (College of Physicians and Surgeons of Manitoba 2007) and noted that in situations where no resolution of con-flicting perspectives involving withdrawing or withholding life sustaining treatment could be achieved, the physician had final authority.

The physicians' decision to transfer Mr. Golubchuk to a palliative care setting was blocked by a legal injunction initi-ated by the family. This injunction instructed the hospital and care team to continue life-supporting care until a more com-prehensive legal review and decision could be provided. The ICU physicians objected, citing the official policy statement and their personal objections to providing care that violated their professional judgment about what constituted appropri-ate, compassionate care. Although a Jewish physician with a background in intensive care medicine agreed to manage Mr. Golubchuk's care, before a formal legal challenge of the Col-lege of Physicians and Surgeons of Manitoba policy statement occurred, the patient died. As such, the statement remains as the primary guide for end-of-life decision practice for physi-cians in Manitoba.

Several groups of stakeholders and experts supported the Golubchuk family in their demand for continuation of mechan-ical ventilation and tube feeding. These supporters included people with disabilities who questioned the unilateral decision-making authority of physicians, and spokespersons for ethno-cultural and religious communities who emphasized the need to engage the patient's and family's religious beliefs forbidding discontinuation of life-supporting treatment. One ethicist com-mented, "there are many, many vulnerable individuals and groups in our community who will be even more marginalized in the course of receiving health care if they're on the receiving end of an assessment utilizing this notion of the minimum goal of life-sustaining treatment" (Webster 2008, 54).[21]

Although this book concerns spiritual rather than formal religious beliefs, the Golubchuk case nonetheless enables us to see the way undergraduate medical students are trained to reflect on nonscientific claims and sensibilities. Medical students were asked to use the case to reflect upon the following questions (Pauls 2011, 2): "If you were the main treating physician in these cases what would you do? Does it make a difference if the patient/their family want to stop (treatment) or if the physician does? What are the good points or positives about the College statement and what are some of the bad points or negatives?"

Tutorial leaders with backgrounds in bioethics and clinical medicine were initially asked to engage the religious/spiritual dimension of the Jewish family's values and resulting legal challenge to the ICU physicians' initial decision to discontinue treatment. Nevertheless, students were advised, "While the family's religious beliefs are a very important element here, they do not mean that treatment must continue" (Pauls 2011, 2).

Moreover, some of the public and medical legal debate centered on the content and specificity of alternative interpretations of Talmudic scholars, who either emphasized the duty to preserve life to the point of actual death or who identified a one-day interval during which people were recognized as dying and where no duty of extraordinary care was required. However, when this case was used with medical students, the undergraduates were instructed: "In the Golubchuk case, the first thing the physician should do is try to reestablish communication with the family, and try to better understand their reasons for wanting to continue [life-supporting care]." "Sometimes people don't fully understand the risks and limitations of the interventions we provide" (Pauls 2011, 2). Students were further informed: "It is also important that the physician explore his or her own reasons for wanting to stop (treatment)" (Pauls 2011, 2). However, no specific references to religious or spiritual dimensions of these "reasons" were included in the teaching materials, even though such forces would likely be at the heart of many physicians' interpretations of this case. In short, while the Golubchuk narrative encourages discussion of whether patients and family members asserting religious or spiritual beliefs have a right to demand all possible treatment interventions, the overarching tendency among the tutors using this case was to establish pragmatic prospects for mediation and reconciliation of conflicting perspectives on end-of-life care treatment decisions.

This example is distinctive because it is grounded in a widely publicized and legally contested case. Moreover, this case might remind us that with regard to conflicts over the provision or discontinuation of life-supporting measures, patients entering hospice palliative care may share the perceptions and experiences of people living with long-term disability, chronic illness, or the challenges of structural or cultural barriers to equitable care. Patients and their families may also be influenced by previous experiences of conflict with care providers in decisions centering on the efficacy or futility of treatment and engagement of their requests for referral or mediation. Indeed, many patients entering hospice care will have been influenced by the media depictions of cases such as this in which care providers appear to be guided most strongly by formal professional ethical and legal policies. For vulnerable people in end-of-life care, the Golubchuk case may reinforce their own perceptions that the health care system promotes a largely formal and instrumental engagement of religion and spirituality.

CONCLUDING REMARKS

In these case studies, we can see a consistent emphasis on a pragmatic and mechanistic problem-solving model of clinical practice. There is nothing inherently inappropriate about this tendency. After all, there are significant pressures on medical schools and residency programs to produce physicians who will provide substantial and efficient benefits to their society and their health care teams within often highly constrained economic, temporal, scientific, and political parameters. Our claim is not that physicians' common instrumentalist approach to the role of spirituality in the lives of their patients reflects a diabolical or heartless approach to human suffering; far from it. Our interest is, rather, in observing both the meta-narratives that appear to govern the way we practice and think about medicine as well as the particular expressions of these accounts. To this end, we have argued that a relatively recent interest in medical humanities has not yet supplanted the "hidden curriculum" in most medical schools that creates a culture of pragmatism in which it is difficult to facilitate serious and substantive reflection on the religious and spiritual dimensions of human health. The hiddenness of this curriculum alone means that it may create unforeseeable obstacles for patients and clinicians.

While in most cases the formal curriculum of medical education is no longer articulated in an explicitly or aggressively hegemonic manner, and while it is clear that the broader non-medical culture in the West has for perhaps two or three decades begun to question the supremacy of the allopathic model, this model continues to be privileged in such a way that religious and spiritual concerns are usually marginal instrumental concerns. Again, this is not the result of some conspiracy on the part of medical educators; rather, it is largely a function of the tendency of entrenched ideologies to be preserved both by their bona fide successes as well as the cumulative weight of their decades (or centuries) of establishment.

It is worthwhile to reflect on the implications of the observations we have made in this chapter for medical students, residents, and physicians engaged in hospice palliative care work—and for the nurses, social workers, family members, and volunteers who work with these caregivers. It is helpful to remember that the hospice movement was initially more identified with nursing, pastoral care, and other disciplines more explicitly engaged with the notion of spirituality. As such, it should not be surprising if in fact those physicians drawn to hospice work are also comparatively more open to or sensitive about the significance of spirituality in the lives of their patients than other medical professionals might be. We have no doubt that this is true, and that this tendency is a great boon to the patients and families involved. However, in order to ensure that hospice palliative caregivers address the religious or spiritual needs of their patients and the concerns of their medial colleagues in an informed manner, it is important for hospice physicians to grapple seriously with the ways that the institutions in which they work and the meta-narratives that legitimate those organizations have influenced the practice of medicine (Byrne 2008). Moreover, in order for hospice palliative caregivers to continue to set an example for other physicians regarding the ways professionals might engage meaningfully in conversations with patients and colleagues about spirituality, it is important to be involved in continually reevaluating the complex and often problematic ways religion and spirituality are framed by physicians and medical educators.

NOTES

1. It is also the case, though, that secularization unfolded and is still unfolding very unevenly in Europe and North America. In some societies, over time religion became constrained by republicanism, leading in the United States to its flourishing and in France to its diminishment. However, in other places such as Canada, where—much to the shock of many Canadians—there has never been a definitive "separation of church and state," the Queen of England ("Supreme Governor" of the Church of England) is still our head of state, religious schools receive some degree of public funding in most provinces, and religiously affiliated hospitals continue to receive public funding, the situation has always been rather mixed.

2. Readers interested in this rapidly growing form of spirituality should consult http://www.sbnr.org/.

3. This meta-narrative is, of course, unidirectional, and in that sense rather misleading. In fact, it may well be that there is a fairly constant level of interest in or "demand" for the ideas, art, experiences, and certainties associated with religion, but that the "suppliers" are no longer a small handful of official religious groups but a much larger collection of religious and spiritual resources (see Stark and Bainbridge 1996).

4. See also the 2010 story of an anesthesiologist charged with sexually molesting patients who were under sedation ("MD facing sex charges subject of 2008 complaint," CBCNews, Sep-

tember 30, 2010, http://www.cbc.ca/news/canada/toronto/story/2010/09/30/doctor-charges.html?ref=rss.

5. See "Dr. Charles Smith: The man behind the public inquiry," CBCNews, April 10, 2010, http://www.cbc.ca/news/canada/story/2009/12/07/f-charles-smith-goudge-inquiry.html.

6. The misdiagnoses occurred in Newfoundland and may have resulted in hundreds of deaths and needless surgeries. See Deana Stokes Sullivan and Gillian Woodford, "Cancer scandal puts path standards under the scope," *National Review of Medicine*, June 15, 2007, 007http://www.nationalreviewofmedicine.com/issue/2007/06_15/4_patients_practice03_11.html.

7. This story relates to the now patently specious claims made over the years by Dr. Andrew Wakefield. His claims had a significant impact on the anti-immunization movement. See "Autism and MMR vaccine controversy," CBCNews, January 7, 2011, http://www.cbc.ca/news/health/story/2011/01/06/f-autism-measles-vaccine-timeline.html.

8. Of course, these scandals are also not exactly new; after all, the infamous Tuskegee syphilis study (1932–1972) involving the intentional infection of hundreds of impoverished African Americans made news in the late 1960s both as an illustration of deep-seated racism and unethical medical practices in the United States.

9. Aijing Shang et al., "Are the clinical effects of homeopathy placebo effects? Comparative study of placebo-controlled trials of homoeopathy and allopathy," *The Lancet* 366 (9487), August 2005: 726–32, http://www.thelancet.com/journals/lancet/article/PIIS0140-6736(05)67177-2/fulltext.

10. Wakefield's 1998 paper showing a link between autism and the MMR vaccine was retracted by *The Lancet*, but not before making a significant impact on the anti-immunization movement. See note 7, "Autism and MMR vaccine controversy."

11. See, for example, the *Journal of Evidence-Based Complementary and Alternative Medicine*, http://www.hindawi.com.ezproxy.library.uvic.ca/journals/ecam/?content/by/year/2008.

12. It is worth noting that Muslim, Sikh, Hindu, and Buddhist

communities nearly doubled or more than doubled in each of the past two decades, while the SBNR subculture has grown in leaps and bounds in especially the past fifteen years. These combined areas of growth appear likely to reshape both the religious and institutional landscape of Canada for the foreseeable future.

13. Indeed, in the case of Bramadat's wife's medical training and residency program (in the late 1990s), these alternative traditions were not covered at all.

14. See Eighteenth International Congress on Palliative Care, October 5–8, 2010, http://www.palliativecare.ca/en/index. html.

15. See McGill Medicine Whole Person Care, http://www. mcgill.ca/wholepersoncare/.

16. George Engel, "The biopsychosocial model and medical education: Who are to be the teachers?" *The New England Journal of Medicine*, April 1, 1982, http://www.nejm.org/ doi/full/10.1056/NEJM198204013061311.

17. See Daniel P. Sulmasy, "A biopsychosocial model for the care of patients at the end of life," *The Gerontologist* 42(3), 2002, http://gerontologist.oxfordjournals.org/content/42/ suppl_3/24.full.

18. The curriculum development data, case studies, and narrative interviews with medical educators and care providers cited in this chapter were collected with the support of a five-year CIHR New Emerging Team Grant: End of Life Care and Vulnerable Populations, 2005–2011 (H. Chochinov, D. Stienstra, Z. Lutfiyya, and J. Kaufert). All personal and identifying details have been altered to protect the anonymity of the informants.

19. Parts of this case were presented in two collections (Kaufert and O'Neil 1995; Kaufert et al. 1999) dealing with cross-cultural issues in death and dying.

20. The case was developed by Sarah Bowen (1995) and used in teaching tutorials in immigrant and refugee reproductive health between 1998 and 2010.

21. While legal precedents clearly support the rights of patients and their proxies to refuse treatment, the law is much less clear about the rights of individuals and families to

demand treatments where there is no clear evidence of benefit or counter evidence that the "life-sustaining treatment" imposed unacceptable harms (Pope 2008).

REFERENCES

Bowen, S. 1995. *Case example for HD006 cross cultural perspectives on reproductive health—versions 1998–2010.* Department of Community Health Sciences, Faculty of Medicine, University of Manitoba.

Bramadat, P., and D. Seljak, eds. 2005. *Religion and ethnicity in Canada.* Toronto: Pearson.

———. 2008. *Christianity and ethnicity in Canada.* Toronto: University of Toronto Press.

Buck, H. 2006. Spirituality: Concept analysis and model development. *Holistic Nursing Practice* 20(6): 288–92.

Byrne, M. 2008. Spirituality in palliative care: What language do we need? *International Journal of Palliative Care Nursing* 14(6): 274–80.

CBCNews. 2011. Autism and MMR vaccine controversy. 7 January. www.cbc.ca. http://www.cbc.ca/news/health/story/2011/01/06/f-autism-measles-vaccine-timeline.html (Accessed February 7, 2011).

Chernish, G. 2010. *Handbook of Complementary Medicine.* Winnipeg: Program in Medical Humanities, Faculty of Medicine, University of Manitoba.

Chiesa, A., and A. Serretti. 2010. A systematic review of neurobiological and clinical features of mindfulness meditations. *Psychological Medicine* 40(8): 1239–52.

Coburn, D., G. Torrance, and J. Kaufert. 1983. Medical dominance in Canada in historical perspective: The rise and fall of medicine? *International Journal of Health Services* 13(3): 407–32.

Code, L. 1991. *What can she know? Feminist theory and the construction of knowledge.* Ithaca, NY: Cornell University Press.

Cohen, M. 1995. Sanctions against sexual abuse of patients by doctors: Sex differences in attitudes among young family physicians. *Canadian Medical Association Journal* (153): 169–76.

The College of Physicians and Surgeons of Manitoba. 2007. Withholding and withdrawing life-sustaining treatment. Statement No. 1602. College of Physicians and Surgeons of Manitoba. http://www.cpsm.mb.ca/index.php.

Coward, H., and P. Ratanakul, eds. 1999. *A cross-cultural dialogue on health care ethics.* Waterloo: Wilfrid Laurier Press.

Engel, G. L. 1977. The need for a new medical model: A challenge for biomedicine. *Science* 196(4286): 129–36.

Goldine, P. R., and J. J. Gross. 2010. Effects of mindfulness-based stress reduction (MBSR) on emotional regulation in social anxiety disorder. *Emotion* 10(1): 83–91.

Holmes, H. B., and L. M. Purdy, eds. 1992. *Feminist perspectives in medical ethics.* Bloomington: Indiana University Press.

Kaufert, J., and J. O'Neil. 1995. Cultural mediation of dying and grieving among native patients in urban hospitals. In *The path ahead: Readings in death and dying*, ed. L. A. DeSpelder and A. Strickland. Mayfield, CA: Mountain View Press, 59–74.

Kaufert, J., and R. Putsch. 1997. Communication through interpreters in health care: Ethical dilemmas arising from differences in class, culture, language and power. *Journal of Clinical Ethics* (8): 7–87.

Kaufert, J., R. W. Putsch, and M. Lavallee. 1999. End-of-life decision making among Aboriginal Canadians: Interpretation, mediation and discord in the communication of bad news. *Journal of Palliative Care* 151: 31–38.

Kaufert, J., et al. 2010. End-of-life ethics and disability: Differing perspectives in case-based teaching. *Medicine, Health Care and Philosophy* 13: 115–26.

Kaufert, J., R. Weibe, M. Lavallee, P. Kaufert. 2012. The experience of Indigenous peoples in accessing hospice care: Seeking physical, cultural, ethical, and spiritual "safe space" for a good death. In *Religious understandings of a good death in hospice palliative care*, ed. H. Coward and K. I. Stajduhar. Albany: State University of New York Press.

Linden, D. E. 2006. How psychotherapy changes the brain: The contribution of functional neuroimaging. *Molecular Psychiatry* 11(6): 528–38.

Magwood, B. 2003. The Medical Humanities Program at the University of Manitoba, Winnipeg Manitoba, Canada. *Academic Medicine* 78(10): 1015–19.

Mayo, K. R. 2009. Support from neurobiology for spiritual techniques for anxiety: A brief review. *Journal of Health Care Chaplaincy* 16(1-2): 53–57.

McBrien, B. 2006. A concept analysis of spirituality. *British Journal of Nursing* 15(1): 42–45.

National Commission for the Protection of Human Subjects of Biomedical and Behavioral Research. 1978. *The Belmont report: Ethical principles and guidelines for the protection of human subjects of research.* Washington, DC: U.S. Department of Health, Education, and Welfare.

Pauls, M. 2011. End of life ethics. Tutorial leader's notes, Program in Medical Humanities, Faculty of Medicine, University of Manitoba. Used with permission.

Pesut, B., et al. 2008. Conceptualizing spirituality and religion for health care. *Journal of Clinical Nursing* 17: 2803–10.

Pope, W. 2008. Summary of the College of Physicians and Surgeons of Manitoba statement on withholding and withdrawing life-sustaining treatment. In *End of life ethics and decision-making: Current policy debates about withholding and withdrawing life-sustaining treatments,* ed. R. Weibe and L. Neufeld. Unpublished conference proceedings from the Canadian Institutes for Health Research Knowledge Translation Forum, Department of Community Health Sciences, University of Manitoba, Winnipeg, June 9, 2008, 17–36.

Ptak, C., and A. Petronis. 2008. Epigenetics and complex disease: From etiology to new therapeutics. *Annual Review of Pharmacology and Toxicology* 48: 257–76.

Seljak, D. 2005. Education, multiculturalism and religion. In *Religion and ethnicity in Canada,* ed. P. Bramadat and D. Seljak. Toronto: Pearson, 178–201.

Shang, A., et al. 2005. Are the clinical effects of homoeopathy placebo effects? Comparative study of placebo-controlled trials of homoeopathy and allopathy. *The Lancet* 336(9487): 726–32. http://www.thelancet.com/journals/lancet/article/PIIS0140-6736(05)67177-2/fulltext (Accessed February 7, 2011).

Sharpley, C. F. 2010. A review of the neurobiological effects of psychotherapy for depression. *Psychotherapy: Theory, Research, Practice, Training* 47(4): 603–15.

Sherwin, S. 1992. *No longer patient: Feminist ethics and health care.* Philadelphia: Temple University Press.

———. 2008. Whither bioethics? How feminism can help reorient bioethics. *International Journal of Feminist Approaches to Bioethics* 1(1): 7–27.

Stephenson, P. 2005. Health care, religion, and ethnic diversity in Canada. In *Religion and ethnicity in Canada*, ed. P. Bramadat and D. Seljak. Toronto: Pearson, 201–21.

Solomon, M. Z. 1997. From what's neutral to what's meaningful: Reflections on a study of medical interpreters. *Journal of Clinical Ethics* 8(1): 88–93.

Stark, R., and W. S. Bainbridge. 1996. *A theory of religion.* New Brunswick, NJ: Rutgers University Press.

Sulmasy, D. P. 2003. A biopsychosocial-spiritual model for the care of patients at the end of life. *The Gerontologist* 42(3): 24–33. http://gerontologist.oxfordjournals.org/content/42/suppl-3/24.full.

Swatos, W., and D. Olson, eds. 2000. *The secularization debate.* Oxford: Rowman & Littlefield.

Taylor, C. 2007. *The secular age.* Boston: Harvard University Press.

Webster, G. 2008. Between a rock and a hard place: Is the CPSM statement an ethical remedy? In *End of life ethics and decision-making: Current policy debates about withholding and withdrawing life-sustaining treatments*, ed. R. Weibe and L. Neufeld. Unpublished conference proceedings from the Canadian Institutes for Health Research Knowledge Translation Forum, Department of Community Health Sciences, University of Manitoba, Winnipeg, June 9, 2008, 52–57.

CHAPTER 4

Research and Practice

Spiritual Perspectives of a Good Death
within Evidence-Based Health Care

SHANE SINCLAIR AND HARVEY MAX CHOCHINOV

INTRODUCTION

SPIRITUAL PERSPECTIVES of a "good death" are constructed
from various faith traditions, philosophies, cultures, and life
experiences. While commonalities exist, the notion of a "good
death" is fashioned during the dying process itself and is
shaped by the quality of care available at the end of life. Spirituality has been formally recognized by health organizations,
professional bodies, and health faculties as an important component of human health, especially at the end of life (World
Health Organization 2007). While these formal endorsements
of spirituality's modifying effects on the dying process validate
clinical interventions as well as empirical research addressing
these issues, an important but often overlooked evidence base is
the experience of patients who are facing the end of life. While
spiritual perspectives and notions of a "good death" abound
in various traditions and fields of scholarship, in this chapter
we argue that the perspectives of patients facing the end of life
and the perspectives of their health care professionals provide
a unique and invaluable perspective on this issue. Although a

number of authors in this volume (especially Garces-Foley and Grant) draw attention to the problematic assumption that spirituality is a universal human experience, we adopt a phenomenological approach to the way these concepts are employed in clinical and academic settings. As such, we employ the terms as they are used within hospice palliative care settings, and in those contexts, the universality of the term "spirituality" is accepted alongside other domains of human health. We ground our discussion within clinical research, with the construct of dignity at the end of life being presented as a potential rhetoric and framework for understanding this ineffable and vitally important topic.

THE ORIGINS AND EVOLUTION OF EMPIRICAL APPROACHES TO SPIRITUALITY WITHIN HEALTH CARE

In order to effectively understand a spiritual perspective of a "good death" within evidence-based health care, an initial understanding of the historical and conceptual factors framing this perspective is necessary. Empiricism, the epistemological foundation of evidence-based health care, is a theory of knowledge within the natural sciences that is based on observation and experimentation rather than intuition or revelation (Webster 1946). The foundational assumption of empiricism is that only one reality exists and that this reality can be observed, measured, validated, and controlled through the senses (Machamer and Silberstein 2002). Empirical interest in the spiritual components of health and a "good death" have evolved from a state of relative nonexistence forty years ago to a burgeoning research field at present (tables 4.1 and 4.2). While the field of religious studies has had a long-standing interest in examining spiritual issues, interest in these matters within health care is a relatively recent phenomenon that is rooted within clinical experience rather than a specific faith tradition. The growth of research on spirituality within health care raises many salient questions, including: What factors have led to such increased

TABLE 4.1.
LITERATURE SEARCH: KEYWORD "SPIRITUAL$" (AS OF DECEMBER 31, 2009)

Periodical Discipline	MEDLINE (Medicine)	CINAHL Plus (Nursing)	ATLA (Religious Studies)
1960–1969	45	9	1,060
1970–1979	183	30	1,930
1980–1989	547	214	4,394
1990–1999	1,724	1,444	7,210
2000–2009	6,000	4,813	8,977
TOTAL	8,499	6,510	23,571

TABLE 4.2.
LITERATURE SEARCH: KEYWORD "GOOD DEATH" (AS OF DECEMBER 31, 2010)

MEDLINE	CINAHL	ATLA
363	1,621	65

Tables 4.1 and 4.2 adapted with permission from S. Sinclair et al., "A Thematic Review of the Spirituality Literature within Palliative Care," *Journal of Palliative Medicine* 9(2): 464–79. © 2006, Mary Ann Liebert, Inc.

activity? and How are spirituality and a "good death" conceptualized within contemporary health care?

A number of theories have been proposed to explain the increased interest in spirituality among various health care disciplines. As Bruce and Stajduhar and Bramadat and Kaufert in this volume each articulate, researchers in both medicine and nursing have had a particular interest in recent years in the application of an empirical approach to this domain. Possible reasons for this include the emergence of qualitative research methods, allowing for the experiential nature of the topic to be empirically studied; the development of a more holistic understanding of health; the emergence of more pluralistic patient populations; an attempt to reintegrate spirituality and health care; and a shift in terminology from "religion" to "spirituality" (Sinclair et al. 2006a). While each of these theories likely contributed to the emergence of the spirituality and health research field, we suggest that the trend is not unique to the health care field, but is indicative of a much larger paradigmatic shift between modern and postmodern thought as the grand narratives of modernity (biomedical science and religion) are being reinterpreted through a more personal and holistic lens (Grant et al. 2010).

SPIRITUAL PERSPECTIVES
IN A PLURALISTIC SOCIETY

Almost fifty years ago, Karl Rahner proclaimed, "the committed believer of tomorrow will either be a 'mystic'—someone who has 'experienced' something—or will not exist anymore" (1971, 15). Data from a recent Canadian census seems to verify Rahner's claim, as a growing number of Canadians seem to primarily identify themselves as spiritual, with religion taking on a secondary role (Bibby 2009). Between 1985 and 2004, the number of Canadians aged fifteen and older who identified as having no religious affiliation increased from 12 percent to 17 percent (Clark and Schellenberg 2006). While religious affiliation comprises only one facet of religiosity (along with attendance, personal practice, and importance), when one considers that 25 percent of Canadians who identified as religious had not attended a religious service in the past year, the significance of this shift becomes more evident. Finally, when the four dimensions of religiosity are aggregated and indexed, 40 percent of Canadians are categorized as having a low degree of religiosity, 31 percent as moderately religious, and 29 percent as highly religious (Clark and Schellenberg 2006). While religiosity has declined, when Canadians were asked, "Do you believe God or a Higher Power exists?" 49 percent responded, "Yes I definitely do," with 33 percent answering, "Yes, I think so," 11 percent answering, "No, I don't think so," and 7 percent answering, "No, I definitely don't" (Bibby 2006). These results seem to suggest that while religiosity has declined in recent decades, Canadians continue to espouse beliefs that are largely self-discovered rather than dogmatically determined. This shift within Canadian society from a religious to a spiritual perspective is underscored by the finding that 54 percent of Canadians acknowledge having spiritual needs, including 25 percent of self-identified atheists (Bibby 2009). This growing group of individuals who see themselves as spiritual but not necessarily religious is further evident in a recent study reporting that when spirituality is defined as a connection with others and finding meaning in life, it is a term that even atheists accept (Smith-Stoner 2007).

While this shift is less pronounced in the United States, a similar trend is unfolding. In 2001, 14 percent of the U.S. population indicated "no religious preference," a twofold increase from the prior decade (Garces-Foley 2006; ARIS 2000). Consistent with Canadian survey data, while only a modest number of respondents explicitly identify themselves as "spiritual but not religious," when religious activity is taken into account, this shift toward a more spiritual orientation is more evident. For example, a U.S. Gallup survey reports that while 47 percent of Americans identify themselves as spiritually committed, only 13 percent strongly agreed with all nine items of the spiritual commitment scale. These results suggest that while Americans see themselves as being spiritually committed, their commitment is largely self-defined and less associated with religious activity (The George H. Gallup International Institute 2003). While survey data suggests that spirituality and religion are distinct concepts, caution needs to be exercised, given that many continue to argue that they are interconnected (Sinclair et al. 2006a; Garces-Foley 2006; Marler and Hadaway 2002).

CONCEPTUALIZATIONS OF SPIRITUALITY WITHIN CLINICAL AND EMPIRICAL HEALTH CARE

Within modern health care, this societal shift has resulted in spirituality and the notion of a good death being largely conceived in secular terms, characterized by inclusivity related to distinctive interpretations of the nature of meaning and purpose; notably, notions of the good death are increasingly distinct from religion. This secular approach to spirituality is evident in a recent article exploring the spiritual dimensions of dying in pluralistic societies. Grant et al. argue that "religions, in Western cultures, are disappearing. . . . Spirituality, though commonly practiced within the framework of religion, can also be experienced outside formal religious structures" (2010, 659). While this claim is contentious, it certainly represents one of the dominant assumptions of health research on religion and spirituality. Moreover, while most health care researchers refrain from prognosticating on the evolving influence of religion in contemporary society, the conceptualization of spirituality and religion as being distinct yet interrelated concepts is common within the field. For instance, a recent consensus project on improving the quality of spiritual care in palliative care defined spirituality as "the aspect of humanity that refers to the way individuals seek and express meaning and purpose and the way they experience their connectedness to the moment, to self, to others, to nature and to the significant or the sacred" (Puchalski et al. 2009, 887). While this highly eclectic, individually defined, and experiential understanding of spirituality is challenged by scholars of religious studies (Rose 2001; Garces-Foley 2006), there are a number of pragmatic factors that have contributed to this understanding that bear further discussion.

The subsuming of religion under the broader rubric of spirituality was influenced by the emergence of spirituality as a separate universal domain of human health within contemporary health care (Burton 1998; Bush and Bruni 2008; Lemmer 2002; McSherry and Draper 1997; Olson et al. 2003; Pesut et al. 2008). Articulating spirituality as a dimension of human health appears to provide clinicians and researchers with a universally applicable empirical framework. While this empirically valid and inclusive approach had many benefits, it resulted in a compartmentalized understanding of spirituality (Walters 2004). While integrative approaches are becoming more common, historically, the concepts of body, mind, and spirit have been treated independently within evidence-based health care. The World Health Organization definition of palliative care further reflects this multidimensional understanding of human health:

> Palliative care is an approach that improves the quality
> of life of patients and their families facing the problems

associated with life-threatening illness, through the pre-
vention and relief of suffering by means of early identification and impeccable assessment and treatment of
pain and other problems, physical, psychosocial and
spiritual. (2007)

Also shaping the conceptualization of spirituality and the
concept of a "good death" within health care are the researchers and research participants involved in such studies. Freedman et al. (2002) conducted a review of the 397 articles in
Larson et al.'s seminal overview of the spirituality and health
literature (Larson et al. 1997). They reported that the papers
cited primarily represented patients who were Caucasian (85
percent), American (73 percent), and Christian (95 percent,
when mentioned), noting that the results may therefore not be
reflective of other cultures, faiths, and worldviews. While the
specific demographics of researchers are difficult to ascertain,
Chiu et al. (2004) surveyed the spirituality literature in health
care, reporting that 79.5 percent of the articles originated in the
United States, with only 2.4 percent of articles originating from
non-Western countries. What has emerged from these studies is
a finite understanding of spirituality as a modifier of illness that
ameliorates disease and associated distress through a formulary
of hope, peace, faith, and meaning (Sinclair et al. 2006a); this
observation echoes the argument (Bramadat and Kaufert, chapter 3 in this book) about the emphasis on an "instrumental"
understanding of religion and spirituality in medical training.
Furthermore, equating spirituality with positive experiences
not only results in a one-sided view of spiritual experience, but
promotes spirituality as a "means for self-interested individuals to attain the nearly universally desirable commodity that is
individual health" (Shuman and Meador 2003, 6).

While the Western hospice and palliative care movement
was largely Christian in origin, as Garces-Foley notes in chapter
1 in this book, it has since adopted a perspective that subsumes
religious and nonreligious perspectives within a broader concept of spirituality (Lee et al. 2004; MacConville 2006). Cicely
Saunders, the founder of the hospice movement, reflected this
sentiment in a letter to a colleague in 1965:

I am interested that religion is never discussed or hardly at all under its own heading but only under the work of the chaplain. . . . I do not mean that in most cases they would ever speak of it directly but communication with words of security based on that dimension is, I think, of immense importance in helping the patient to find his own meaning. (2002, 95)

While this inclusive person-centered approach has been criticized as "misty, evanescent, wispy and rich in appeal to narcissism" (Marty 1996, 439) and is often unfairly juxtaposed with religion, we suggest that this approach was primarily influenced by the perspectives of dying individuals and the subsequent clinical experiences of their health care professionals, rather than a particular agenda on the part of palliative care clinicians and researchers.

THE IMPORTANCE OF SPIRITUALITY AND THE SPIRITUAL PERSPECTIVE OF PATIENTS

While there remains a lack of consensus regarding the precise nature of spirituality and its relationship to related fields of religion, existentialism, quality of life, and psychosocial issues, the importance of spirituality to patients facing a life-threatening illness is now well established (Puchalski 2002; Steinhauser et al. 2000). Despite the deeply personal nature of spirituality, survey data indicates that the majority of patients express a desire to have their health care professional inquire about their spirituality (Sulmasy 2006). While religious leaders and community visitors represent an important cadre of spiritual care providers, a recent study asked patients to identify individuals they considered to have provided them spiritual care. Religious visitors were identified in 17 percent of cases, with family and friends (41 percent) and clinicians (29 percent) being identified almost twice as frequently (Daaleman et al. 2008). While patients desire to have their spirituality addressed during their dying process, clinicians and health care systems seem reticent to do so. A recent study of a leading U.S. cancer center reported that 75 percent of patients felt that their spiritual needs were not met during a recent hospital admission (Balboni et al. 2007). Alcorn et al. (2010) conducted a study investigating the importance of religion and spirituality among sixty-eight patients with advanced cancer. While 56 percent of patients identified themselves as very or moderately religious, 72 percent considered themselves to be very or moderately spiritual, with 78 percent reporting that religion and/or spirituality had been important in their cancer experience. As Will, Bruce, Stajduhar, and Bramadat and Kaufert articulate in each of their chapters in this volume, addressing the spiritual needs of patients is now being incorporated into the scope of practice of a number of health care disciplines. While health care systems and organizations have also responded to this growing need through the development of multifaith spiritual care programs, their use and integration within these settings presents an ongoing challenge (Sinclair et al. 2009).

While the importance of spirituality to a "good death" has long been attested to by researchers, clinicians, health organizations, and patients themselves, a more challenging issue is determining the spiritual needs of patients facing the end of life and their relationship to a "good death." A study of advanced cancer patients identified the greatest spiritual needs of participants as: 1) overcoming fears (51 percent); 2) finding hope (42 percent); 3) discovering meaning in life (40 percent); and 4) a desire to talk to someone about finding peace (43 percent), meaning in life (28 percent), and death and dying (25 percent) (Moadel et al. 1999). Wright reported similar findings in a study exploring the spiritual needs of palliative care patients in the United Kingdom (2001). The most frequently identified spiritual needs reported were: someone to listen (89 percent), concern for relatives (88 percent), and someone to "be there" (86 percent). The George H. Gallup International Institute conducted a survey that reported on the spiritual needs that patients sought to be addressed by their health care professional (1997). Patients identified the following needs: to have a warm relationship with their providers, to be listened to, to have someone to share their fears and concerns with, to have someone with them in their dying process, to engage in prayer, and to say goodbye to loved ones. Similar results were reported in a study of an interdisciplinary palliative care team, which identified spirituality as a relational process between team members and their patients, often being embedded within acts of caring and routine patient interaction (Sinclair et al. 2006b). Finally, Daaleman et al. (2008) reported on the core components of spiritual care delivery among a group of individuals (clinician and nonclinician) that palliative patients identified as being most involved in their spiritual care. The three core elements of spiritual care delivery were 1) being present; 2) a recognition of the shared humanness between practitioner and patient; and 3) a process termed "co-creating," whereby aspects of patients' spirituality were incorporated into the care plan. While addressing spiritual needs often involves the administration of standardized instruments, spiritual care interventions, and practices, the most important needs according to patients primarily relate to the intrinsic qualities of their health care professionals rather than a specific task, practice, or technique.

THE EFFECT OF SPIRITUALITY ON
QUALITY OF LIFE WITHIN PALLIATIVE CARE

Attention to spirituality at the end of one's life has been demonstrated to be a powerful modifier of quality of life. Quality of life is an important component of a "good death," encompassing the holistic health needs of individuals and their impact on the whole person. The McGill Quality of Life Questionnaire is a multidimensional assessment tool with strong psychometrics, designed to measure quality of life in patients facing the end of life. The questionnaire's existential subscale has consistently demonstrated that existential or spiritual issues are at least as important as other subscales (physical symptoms, psychological symptoms, and support) in predicting overall quality of life (Cohen et al. 1996). Singer reported similar findings in an extensive qualitative study investigating the important domains of end-of-life care for cancer patients (Singer et al. 1999). These included: 1) receiving adequate pain and symptom management; 2) avoiding inappropriate prolongation of dying;

3) achieving a sense of spiritual peace; 4) relieving burdens; and 5) strengthening relationships with loved ones. Working at the end of life was recently reported to have a largely positive impact on the spiritual lives of health care professionals, suggesting that despite the many challenges at the end of life, there are also numerous benefits (Sinclair 2011).

Kuhl found spiritual/existential issues to be as important as biomedical needs among a heterogeneous sample of patients facing the end of life (2002). Another study reported that spiritual well-being was significantly associated with an ability of cancer patients to enjoy life, despite high levels of pain or fatigue (Brady et al. 1999). In a separate study, existential/spiritual factors (e.g., maintaining one's dignity, feeling prepared to die) were identified as being important to patients, family members, physicians, and health care providers (Steinhauser et al. 2000). While there was consensus among the four groups in this study, a number of spiritual factors were rated as important by patients, but not physicians, including being at peace with God (89 percent vs. 65 percent), prayer (85 percent vs. 55 percent), and feeling one's life is complete (80 vs. 58 percent). Related factors deemed important by patients included having someone to listen (95 percent); trusting one's physician (94 percent); maintaining a sense of humor (93 percent); having a physician with whom one can discuss fears (90 percent); having a physician who knows one as a whole person (88 percent); and believing family is prepared for one's death (85 percent). While these factors arguably fall within the realm of bedside etiquette, communication skills, and professionalism, when spirituality is broadly construed in terms of connection and presence, the impact that health care professionals have on patients' spiritual well-being is difficult to deny (Sinclair 2011).

EMPIRICAL MEASURES OF PATIENT SPIRITUALITY

While the spiritual roots of the hospice movement were anchored in the Christian tradition, the universal perspective on spirituality that has developed includes religious and non-religious perspectives, providing a framework to effectively address and measure the diverse spiritual needs of all patients (Sinclair et al. 2006a; Breitbart 2002; Vanistendael 2007). This inclusive approach to spirituality is further evident within spiritual assessments designed to measure different aspects of patient spirituality (Selman et al. 2010; Fitchett and Handzo 1998; Mystakidou et al. 2007; Peterman et al. 2002; Tamura et al. 2006; Vivat 2008). A recent systematic review identified eighty-five measures of spirituality, with thirty-eight being utilized specifically within palliative care (Selman et al. 2010). An inherent challenge in the design of these instruments is determining the precise relationship between the existential and religious factors. The Spiritual Belief Inventory, for example, while using the term "spiritual" in its title, is technically a measure of religion, given that ten of the fifteen items measure religious practice and belief, while the remaining five items measure support from one's religious community (Holland et al. 1998). In contrast, the FACIT Spiritual Well-Being Scale provides a cumulative score on the overarching construct of spirituality based on two subscales—one corresponding to faith and the other to meaning/peace (Fitchett and Handzo 1998). While spiritual assessments provide clinicians and researchers with the tools to both assess and measure spiritual issues, they are also problematic as they attempt to quantify a seemingly ineffable force through empirical means. A further challenge facing spiritual assessments is their emphasis on positive outcomes, which invariably equate the absence of these attributes with a low level of spirituality.

SPIRITUAL DISTRESS

A consensus project on improving the quality of palliative care recently recommended the routine and ongoing screening for spiritual distress (Puchalski et al. 2009). Spiritual distress pertains to a range of issues including meaninglessness, hopelessness, religious beliefs, forgiveness, demoralization, continuity of self, and spiritual comfort, which respondents rate on a Likert scale (Hui et al. 2011; Selman et al. 2010; Puchalski et al. 2009). Spiritual distress is prevalent among patients facing the end of life, with 44 percent of patients in a recent study meeting the criteria for spiritual distress, particularly those who were young, experiencing pain, and suffering from depression (Hui et al. 2011). A separate study exploring the prevalence of spiritual pain in advanced cancer patients revealed that 96 percent of participants reported having had spiritual pain in their lifetime, with 61 percent identifying spiritual pain at the time of the study (Mako et al. 2009). The following seven domains of spiritual distress, while difficult to diagnose and differentiate from psychosocial distress, are identified by Hui et al. (2011): hope vs. despair; wholeness vs. brokenness; courage vs. anxiety/dread; connection vs. alienation; meaningful vs. meaningless; grace/forgiveness vs. guilt; and empowered vs. helpless. Spirituality, particularly when it is understood as the pursuit of meaning and purpose, has also been shown to have a significant impact in warding off certain aspects of distress (Chochinov et al. 2009). A separate study demonstrated a negative association between spirituality and religiosity and depressive symptoms (Nelson et al. 2002), while Wilson et al. reported that religious beliefs were negatively correlated to requests for hastened death (2007).

Spiritual distress represents a significant threat to predictors of a "good death." Its impact is even more pronounced among patients expressing a desire for a hastened death. While desire for a hastened death has been reported in 7 to 9 percent of patients with advanced disease, the prevalence of desire for hastened death increases significantly among patients experiencing depression, hopelessness, and meaninglessness (Wilson et al. 2007; Jones et al. 2003; Thompson and Chochinov 2010). While there is a strong association between depression and desire for hastened death, the experience of hopelessness was identified as an even greater predictor of suicidal ideation among the terminally ill (Chochinov et al. 1998). McClain et al. reported that terminally ill cancer patients with good family supports and moderate levels of spiritual well-being were less likely to express a desire for hastened death (2003). Similar findings are evident from the state of Oregon, which has collected patient data from individuals choosing to end their life by physician-assisted suicide (Department of Human Services 2009; Sullivan et al. 2000). As in previous years, patients who chose to end their life in this manner did so for the following reasons: 1) loss of autonomy (96.6 percent); 2) loss of dignity (91.5 percent); and 3) decreasing ability to participate in activities that made life enjoyable (86.4 percent) (Department of Human Services 2009). Physical symptoms, such as inadequate pain control (10.2 percent), played an important, but secondary, role to issues that were related to psychological or spiritual distress.

A study exploring the relationship between desire for hastened death, cancer pain, and depression revealed moderate correlations between desire for hastened death and poor spiritual and religious well-being (Mako et al. 2009). While patients who identify spirituality as an important feature in their life are less likely to experience symptoms that erode a "good death," the impact of spirituality on a "good death" is most pronounced in those whose spiritual well-being is fractured or absent. When spiritual distress is addressed at the end of life, quality of life, well-being, and will to live are maintained and in some instances enhanced. When the spiritual needs of individuals are not attended to, some patients perceive a hastened death as the only viable way out.

DIGNITY AS A MODIFIER OF A "GOOD DEATH"

The construct of dignity is of particular relevance to discussions of spirituality and the end of life. Historically, dignity arose out of the Jewish and Christian notions of being made in the image of God (Barilan 2009) and continues to be a prominent feature of declarations of human rights (Hayry 2004; Harmon 2009). Empirical research has identified dignity as an essential ingredient of a "good death." The essential relationship between the construct of dignity and the notion of a "good death" is often raised within the euthanasia and assisted suicide debate. As Pullman summarized, "Indeed it is not uncommon to find those on either side of an ethical debate invoking some consideration of human dignity in support of their contrary conclusions" (2004, 171). Philosophical differences notwithstanding, most important are the psychosocial and spiritual issues that under-pin considerations for a hastened death. It appears that when dignity is upheld at the end of life, ethical dilemmas related to the right to die are far less likely to surface. Besides influencing desire for hastened death, attending to dignity-related concerns has been shown to mitigate distress leading to such requests (Chochinov et al. 2002).

For the majority of palliative care patients, a sense of dig-nity is maintained throughout the end of life. The importance of dignity, however, is particularly evident when it is fractured or eroded, since dignity is the most frequently cited reason patients give for considering euthanasia or suicide (Sullivan et al. 2000; Meier et al. 1998; Pannuti and Tanneberger 1993). Thus, loss of dignity plays a prominent role in desire for has-tened death. The maintenance of dignity has also been shown to have a powerful effect on diminishing depression, hopeless-ness, and meaninglessness, which are significant barriers to a "good death" (Payne et al. 1996). In short, when dignity is addressed at the end of life, the likelihood of achieving a "good death" is markedly enhanced (Chochinov 2006).

THE DIGNITY MODEL: AN EMPIRICAL PERSPECTIVE ON "GOOD DEATH"

While the importance of dignity in relation to a good death is well established, a more challenging issue is determining specific factors that contribute to an individual's overall sense of dig-nity. The programmatic research of Chochinov and colleagues (Chochinov et al. 2002, 2006, 2008, and 2009; McClement et al. 2004 and 2007; Thompson and Chochinov 2010) has examined these issues, leading to the formation of an empiri-cally derived model of dignity (table 4.3). This model, based on semi-structured interviews with terminally ill patients, identi-fied three major categories related to dignity at the end of life: illness-related concerns, the dignity-conserving repertoire, and the social dignity inventory. Within the dignity model, items related to spirituality are best interpreted within a holistic framework, thereby expanding their application to comprehen-sive palliative care.

TABLE 4.3
MAJOR DIGNITY CATEGORIES, THEMES, AND SUBTHEMES

Illness-related Concerns	Dignity-conserving Repertoire	Social Dignity Inventory
Level of independence	Dignity-conserving perspectives	Privacy boundaries
• Cognitive acuity	• Continuity of self	
• Functional capacity	• Role preservation	Social support
• Symptom distress	• Generativity/legacy	
• Physical distress	• Maintenance of pride	Care tenor
• Psychological distress	• Hopefulness	
• *medical uncertainty*	• Autonomy/control	Burden to others
	• Acceptance	
	• Resilience/fighting spirit	
• *death anxiety*	**Dignity-conserving practices**	Aftermath concerns
	• Living in the moment	
	• Maintaining normalcy	
	• Seeking spiritual comfort	

Reprinted with permission from *Social Science & Medicine*, H. M. Chochinov, T. Hack, S. McClement, L. Kristjanson, and M. Harlos, "Dignity in the Terminally Ill: A Developing Empirical Model," *Social Science & Medicine* 54(43): 3–43. ©2002 Elsevier.

In a subsequent study seeking to validate the dignity model, the feeling that life no longer had meaning or purpose was identified as the only variable that predicted overall sense of dignity (Chochinov et al. 2006), while 87.1 percent of patients indicated that "not being treated with respect" and "feeling a burden to others" were affiliated with their sense of dignity. The dignity-conserving repertoire consists of psychological and spiritual factors patients consider important to their overall sense of dignity (Chochinov 2002). The dignity-conserving repertoire contains two themes, dignity-conserving practices (personal approaches or techniques) and dignity-conserving perspectives (internal qualities and resources) that can be utilized by patients to maintain or enhance their sense of dignity. Dignity-conserving perspectives and practices related to spirituality may be expressed in a number of ways and include continuity of self, generativity/legacy, hopefulness, acceptance, resilience/fighting spirit, acceptance, living "in the moment," and seeking spiritual comfort (Chochinov et al. 2004).

THE PATIENT DIGNITY INVENTORY: AN EMPIRICAL MEASURE FOR THE ENHANCEMENT OF A GOOD DEATH

The Patient Dignity Inventory (PDI) is a twenty-five-item screening tool designed to assess dignity-related distress (table 4.4) (Chochinov et al. 2008). The PDI provides clinicians with a valid, reliable, and novel means of identifying multiple sources of distress in patients facing a life-threatening illness. A factor analysis of the PDI resulted in five factors, including symptom distress, existential distress, dependency, peace of mind, and social support. Factors labeled existential distress (e.g., not feeling like who I once was, not feeling worthwhile or valued, a change in appearance, not being able to carry out important roles, feeling life no longer has meaning, and feeling a burden) and forces eroding peace of mind (e.g., not having made a meaningful contribution, feelings of unfinished business, and concern about spiritual life), while overlapping with the psychosocial domain, seem to be particularly relevant to a spiritual perspective of a "good death."

An additional study used the Patient Dignity Inventory in order to describe the landscape of distress among 253 terminally ill patients (Chochinov et al. 2009). On average, participants identified 5.74 problems, reflecting a variety of physical, psychological, existential, and spiritual issues. Factors associated with specific kinds of distress included being an inpatient, being educated, being younger, and having a partner. Patients also completed the FACIT-SP in order to measure the relationship between PDI items and factors related to spirituality. Eighteen of the twenty-five PDI items were significantly correlated with the total FACIT-SP score, with an overall negative association between the total FACIT-SP scores and the number of PDI items rated as problematic. Compared with the faith subscale, the FACIT-SP meaning and peace subscale was more closely associated with lower levels of distress, suggesting that the experiential effects of spirituality (feeling at peace or having a sense of meaning or purpose) are of more importance than religiosity or a prescribed belief system in mitigating distress.

TABLE 4.4
PATIENT DIGNITY INVENTORY

For each item, please indicate how much of a problem or concern these have been for you within the last few days.	Not a problem	A slight problem	A problem	A major problem	An overwhelming problem
1. Not being able to carry out tasks associated with daily living (e.g., washing myself, getting dressed).	1	2	3	4	5
2. Not being able to attend to my bodily functions independently (e.g., needing assistance with toileting-related activities).	1	2	3	4	5
3. Experiencing physically distressing symptoms (such as pain, shortness of breath, nausea).	1	2	3	4	5
4. Feeling that how I look to others has changed significantly.	1	2	3	4	5
5. Feeling depressed.	1	2	3	4	5
6. Feeling anxious.	1	2	3	4	5
7. Feeling uncertain about my health and health care.	1	2	3	4	5
8. Worrying about my future.	1	2	3	4	5
9. Not being able to think clearly.	1	2	3	4	5
10. Not being able to continue with my usual routines.	1	2	3	4	5
11. Feeling like I am no longer who I was.	1	2	3	4	5
12. Not feeling worthwhile or valued.	1	2	3	4	5
13. Not being able to carry out important roles (e.g., spouse, parent).	1	2	3	4	5
14. Feeling that life no longer has meaning or purpose.	1	2	3	4	5
15. Feeling that I have not made a meaningful and/or lasting contribution in my life.	1	2	3	4	5
16. Feeling that I have "unfinished business" (e.g., things that I have yet to say or do, or that feel incomplete).	1	2	3	4	5
17. Concern that my spiritual life is not meaningful.	1	2	3	4	5

TABLE 4.4 (continued)

For each item, please indicate how much of a problem or concern these have been for you within the last few days.	Not a problem	A slight problem	A problem	A major problem	An overwhelming problem
18. Feeling that I am a burden to others.	1	2	3	4	5
19. Feeling that I don't have control over my life.	1	2	3	4	5
20. Feeling that my health and care needs have reduced my privacy.	1	2	3	4	5
21. Not feeling supported by my community of friends and family.	1	2	3	4	5
22. Not feeling supported by my health care providers.	1	2	3	4	5
23. Feeling like I am no longer able to mentally cope with challenges to my health.	1	2	3	4	5
24. Not being able to accept the way things are.	1	2	3	4	5
25. Not being treated with respect or understanding by others.	1	2	3	4	5

Reprinted with permission from *Journal of Pain and Symptom Management*, H. M. Chochinov, T. Hassard, S. McClement, T. Hack, L. Kristjanson, M. Harlos, S. Sinclair, and A. Murray, "The Patient Dignity Inventory: A Novel Way of Measuring Dignity-Related Distress in Palliative Care," *Journal of Pain and Symptom Management* 36(6): 3–43. © 2008 Elsevier.

THE CARE TENOR: THE IMPACT OF HEALTH CARE PROVIDERS ON DIGNITY AND A GOOD DEATH

An often overlooked factor that influences patients' sense of dignity and the possibility of a "good death" are health care providers working at the patient's bedside. As previously noted, the single most highly endorsed item patients identified as affecting their overall sense of dignity was "not being treated with respect or understanding" (87.1 percent) (Chochinov et al. 2006). While difficult to measure and often ignored, the presence or care tenor that health care providers convey in their interactions with patients has a potentially profound and enduring effect on the individual's sense of dignity. Numerous studies have identified health care providers' qualities such as compassion, kindness, humanity, respect, and empathy as being equally important, or in some instances more important, than professional knowledge or skills (Bush and Bruni 2008; Puchalski 2002; Sulmasy 2006; Sinclair et al. 2006a).

While the Patient Dignity Inventory and other prescriptive measures that assess spiritual distress provide the necessary language to address this important domain, these therapeutic approaches are significantly enhanced by a care tenor that acknowledges dying individuals as persons and not just patients. While spiritual care professionals possess an advanced skill set in the provision of spiritual care (VandeCreek and Burton 2001), recent research has demonstrated that the ABCDs of Dignity Conserving Care (attitudes, behavior, compassion, and dialogue) represent the essential ingredients of the care tenor—aspects of care that fall within the scopes of practice of all health care providers (Chochinov 2007).

CONCLUSION

Empirical research exploring the relationship between spirituality and health has evolved from relative obscurity to a thriving field of scholarly inquiry. Within evidence-based health care, spirituality is generally considered to be a universal dimension of human health, which is individually determined and expressed through nonreligious and religious means. Spirituality, as defined by the individual patient, has also been shown to have a positive effect on factors associated with a "good death." While an underlying discourse has developed within the health care literature, understandings and experiences of spirituality and a "good death" within clinical practice are as diverse as the individuals facing the end of life. While the relationship between spirituality and health care may at times seem vague, and while (as Garces-Foley's chapter establishes) it may be problematic to juxtapose it too simply against religion, a convincing body of evidence has emerged that clearly attests to the significance of one or another form of spirituality to patients' experiences of a "good death." Whatever spiritual perspective patients embrace, spirituality appears to enhance the possibility of a "good death" while buffering factors that erode it. While empirical evidence provides important data demonstrating the influence of spirituality in achieving a "good death," the most compelling evidence comes from the dying themselves, who consistently identify spirituality as vital to their end-of-life experience.

REFERENCES

Alcorn, S. R., M. J. Balboni, H. G. Prigerson, A. Reynolds, A. C. Phelps, A. A. Wright, S. D. Block, J. R. Peteet, L. A. Kachnic, and T. A. Balboni. 2010. If God wanted me yesterday, I wouldn't be here today: Religious and spiritual themes in patients' experiences of advanced cancer. *Journal of Palliative Medicine* 13(5): 581–88.

ARIS. 2000. *American religious identification survey*. New York: The Graduate Center of the City University of New York.

Balboni, T., L. C. Vanderwerker, S. D. Block, E. Paulk, C. S. Lathan, J. R. Peteet, and H. G. Prigerson. 2007. Religiousness and spiritual support among advanced cancer patients and associations with end-of-life treatment preferences and quality of life. *Journal of Clinical Oncology* 25(5): 555–60.

Barilan, Y. M. 2009. From imago dei in the Jewish-Christian traditions to human dignity in contemporary Jewish law. *Kennedy Institute of Ethics Journal* 19(3): 231–59.

Barnard, C. N. 1973. A good death. *Family Health* 5(4): 40–42.

Bibby, R. 2006. *The boomer factor: What Canada's most famous generation is leaving behind*. Toronto: Bastian Books.

———. 2009. *The emerging millennials: How Canada's newest generation is responding to change and choice*. Lethbridge: Project Canada Books.

Boston, P., and B. M. Mount. 2006. The caregiver's perspective on existential and spiritual distress in palliative care. *Journal of Pain and Symptom Management* 32(1): 13–26.

Brady, M. J., A. H. Peterman, G. Fitches, M. Mo, and D. Cella. 1999. A case for including spirituality in quality of life measurement in oncology. *Psycho-Oncology* 8(5): 417–28.

Breitbart, W. 2002. Spirituality and meaning in supportive care: Spirituality and meaning-centered group psychotherapy interventions in advanced cancer. *Supportive Care in Cancer* 10: 272–80.

Burton, L. A. 1998. The spiritual dimension of palliative care. *Seminars in Oncology Nursing* 14(2): 121–8.

Bush, T., and N. Bruni. 2008. Spiritual care as a dimension of holistic care: A relational interpretation. *International Journal of Palliative Nursing* 14(11): 539–45.

Chiu, L., J. D. Emblen, L. Van Hofwegen, R. Sawatzky, and H. Meyerhoff. 2004. An integrative review of the concept of spirituality in the health sciences. *Western Journal of Nursing Research* 26(4): 405–28.

Chochinov, H. M. 2002. Dignity conserving care: A new model for palliative care. *Journal of the American Medical Association* 287(17): 2253–60.

———. 2006. Dying, dignity, and new horizons in palliative end-of-life care. *CA* 56(2): 84–103.

———. 2007. Dignity and the essence of medicine: The A, B, C, and D of dignity conserving care. *British Medical Journal* 335: 184–87.

Chochinov, H. M., T. Hack, T. Hassard, L. J. Kristjanson, S.

McClement, and M. Harlos. 2002. Dignity in the terminally ill: A cross-sectional cohort study. *The Lancet* 360: 2026–30.

Chochinov, H. M., T. Hack, S. McClement, L. Kristjanson, and M. Harlos. 2002. Dignity in the terminally ill: A developing empirical model. *Social Science & Medicine* 54: 433–43.

———. 2004. Dignity and psychotherapeutic considerations in end-of-life care. *Journal of Palliative Care* 20(3): 134–42.

Chochinov, H. M., T. Hassard, S. McClement, T. Hack, L. Kristjanson, M. Harlos, S. Sinclair, and A. Murray. 2008. The patient dignity inventory: A novel way of measuring dignity-related distress in palliative care. *Journal of Pain and Symptom Management* 36(6): 559–71.

———. 2009. The landscape of distress in the terminally ill. *Journal of Pain and Symptom Management* 38(5): 641.

Chochinov, H. M., L. Kristjanson, T. Hack, T. Hassard, S. McClement, and M. Harlos. 2006. Dignity in the terminally ill: Revisited. *Journal of Palliative Medicine* 9(3): 666–72.

Chochinov, H. M., K. G. Wilson, M. Enns, and S. Lander. 1998. Depression, hopelessness, and suicidal ideation in the terminally ill. *Psychosomatics* 39: 366–70.

Clark, W., and G. Schellenberg. 2006. Who's religious? *Canadian Social Trends—Statistics Canada* 11: 2–9.

Cohen, S. R., B. M. Mount, J. J. Tomas, and L. F. Mount. 1996. Existential well-being is an important determinant of quality of life: Evidence from the McGill Quality of Life Questionnaire. *Palliative Medicine* 77: 576–86.

Daaleman, T. P., B. Usher, S. Williams, J. Rawlings, and L. Hanson. 2008. An exploratory study of spiritual care at the end of life. *Annals of Family Medicine* 6(5): 406–11.

De Jong, J. D., and L. E. Clarke. 2009. What is a good death? Stories from palliative care. *Journal of Palliative Care* 25(1): 61–67.

Department of Human Services. 2009. *2009 summary of the state of Oregon's Death with Dignity Act*. State of Oregon, http://www.oregon.gov/DHS/ph/pas/docs/year12.pdf.

Emanuel, E. J., and L. L. Emanuel. 1998. The promise of a good death. *The Lancet* 351(2): SII 21.

Field, M. J., and C. K. Cassel, eds. 1997. *Approaching death: Improving care at the end of life.* Washington, DC: National Academy Press.

Fitchett, G., and G. Handzo. 1998. Spiritual assessment, screening, and intervention. In *Psycho-Oncology*, ed. J. C. Holland. New York: Oxford University Press, 808.

Freedman, O., S. Orenstein, P. Boston, T. Amour, and B. M. Mount. 2002. Spirituality, religion, and health: A critical appraisal of the Larson reports. *The Annals of the Royal College of Physicians and Surgeons of Canada* 35(2): 90–93.

Gallup, G. 1997. *The George H. Gallup International Institute: Spiritual beliefs and the dying process: A report on a national survey.* Princeton: Princeton Religion and Research Center.

Garces-Foley, K. 2006. Hospice and the politics of spirituality. *Omega* 53(1-2): 117–36.

The George H. Gallup International Institute. 2003. *Americans' spiritual searches turn inward.* http://www.gallup.com/poll/7759/americans-spiritual-searches-turn-inward.aspx.

Glavin, B. J., R. A. Engelberg, L. Downey, and J. R. Curtis. 2008. Using the medical record to evaluate the quality of end-of-life care in the intensive care unit. *Critical Care Medicine* 36(4): 1138–46.

Grant, L., S. A. Murray, and A. Sheikh. 2010. Spiritual dimensions of dying in pluralist societies. *British Medical Journal* 341: 659–62.

Harmon, S. 2009. Of plants and people. *European Molecular Biology Organization Reports* 10(9): 946–48.

Hayry, M. 2004. Another look at dignity. *Cambridge Quarterly of Health Care Ethics* 13: 7–14.

Holland, J. C., K. M. Kash, S. D. Passik, M. K. Gronert, A. Sison, M. Lederberg, S. M. Russak, L. Baider, and B. Fox. 1998. A brief spiritual beliefs inventory for use in quality of life research in life-threatening illness. *Psycho-Oncology* 7(6): 460–69.

Hui, D., M. de la Cruz, S. Thorney, H. A. Parsons, M. Delgado-Guay, and E. Bruera. 2011. The frequency and correlates of spiritual distress among patients with advanced cancer admitted to an acute palliative care unit. *American Journal of Hospice and Palliative Medicine* 28: 264–70.

Jones, J. M., M. A. Huggins, A. C. Rydall, and G. M. Rodin. 2003. Symptomatic distress, hopelessness, and the desire for hastened death in hospitalized cancer patients. *Journal of Psychosomatic Research* 55: 411–18.

Karlsson, M., A. Milberg, and P. Strang. 2006. Dying with dignity according to Swedish medical students. *Supportive Care in Cancer* 14(4): 334–39.

Kuhl, D. 2002. *What dying people want.* Toronto: Anchor.

Larson, D. B., J. P. Swyers, and M. E. McCullough. 1997. *Scientific research on spirituality and health: A consensus report.* Rockville, MD: National Institute for Health Care Research.

Lee, V., S. R. Cohen, L. Edgar, A. M. Laizner, and A. J. Gagnon. 2004. Clarifying 'meaning' in the context of cancer research: A systematic literature review. *Palliative and Supportive Care* 2: 291–303.

Lemmer, C. 2002. Teaching the spiritual dimension of nursing care: A survey of U.S. baccalaureate nursing programs. *Journal of Nursing Education* 41(11): 482–90.

Lyotard, J. F. 1979. *The postmodern condition: A report on knowledge,* Trans. G. Bennington and B. Massumi. Minneapolis: University of Minnesota Press.

MacConville, U. 2006. Mapping religion and spirituality in an Irish palliative care setting. *Omega* 53(1-2): 137–52.

Machamer, P. K., and M. Silberstein. (2002). *The Blackwell guide to the philosophy of science.* Oxford: Blackwell Publishers.

Mako, C., K. Galek, and S. Poppito. 2009. Spiritual pain among patients with advanced cancer in palliative care. *Journal of Palliative Medicine* 9(5): 1106–13.

Marler, P. L., and C. K. Hadaway. 2002. 'Being religious' or 'being spiritual' in America: A zero-sum proposition? *Journal for the Scientific Study of Religion* 41(2): 289–300.

Marty, M. E. 1996. Getting organized. *Christian Century* 113(13): 439.

McClain, C. S., B. Rosenfeld, and W. Breitbart. 2003. Effect of spiritual well-being on end-of-life despair in terminally-ill cancer patients. *The Lancet* 361: 1603–7.

McClement, S., H. M. Chochinov, T. Hack, L. J. Kristjanson, and M. Harlos. 2004. Dignity-conserving care: Application of research findings to practice. *International Journal of Palliative Nursing* 10 (4): 173–79.

———. 2007. Dignity therapy: Family member perspectives. *Journal of Palliative Medicine* 10(5): 1076–82.

McSherry, W., and P. Draper. 1997. The spiritual dimension: Why the absence within nursing curricula? *Nurse Education Today* 17(5): 413–17.

Meier, D. E., C. A. Emmons, S. Wallenstein, S. Wallenstein, T. Quill, R. S. Morrison, and C. K. Cassel. 1998. A national survey of physician-assisted suicide and euthanasia in the United States. *New England Journal of Medicine* 338(17): 1193–201.

Miyashita, M., T. Morita, K. Sato, K. Hirai, S. Yasuo, and Y. Uchitomi. 2008. Good death inventory: A measure for evaluating good death from the bereaved family member's perspective. *Journal of Pain and Symptom Management* 35(4): 486–98.

Moadel, A., C. Morgan, A. Fatone, J. Grennan, J. Carter, G. Laruffa, A. Skummy, and J. Dutcher. 1999. Seeking meaning and hope: Self-reported spiritual and existential needs among an ethnically-diverse cancer patient population. *Psycho-Oncology* 8(5): 378.

Mystakidou, K., E. Tsilika, E. Parpa, M. Smyrnioti, and L. Vlahos. 2007. Assessing spirituality and religiousness in advanced cancer patients. *American Journal of Hospice and Palliative Medicine* 23(6): 457–63.

Nelson, C., B. Rosenfield, and W. Breitbart. 2002. Spirituality, religion and depression in the terminally ill. *Psychosomatics* 43: 213–20.

Olson, J. K., P. Paul, L. Douglass, M. B. Clark, J. Simington, and N. Goddard. 2003. Addressing the spiritual dimension in Canadian undergraduate nursing education. *Canadian Journal of Nursing Research* 35(3): 94–107.

Pannuti, F., and S. Tanneberger. 1993. Dying with dignity: Illusion, hope, or human right? *World Health Forum* 14: 172–73.

Payne, S. A., A. Langley-Evans, and R. Hillier. 1996. Perceptions of a "good" death: A comparative study of the views of hospice staff and patients. *Palliative Medicine* 10(307): 312.

Pesut, B., M. Fowler, E. J. Taylor, S. Reimer-Kirkham, and R. Sawatzky. 2008. Conceptualising spirituality and religion for health care. *Journal of Clinical Nursing* 17: 2803–10.

Peterman, A. H., G. Fitches, M. J. Brady, L. Hernandez, and D. Cella. 2002. Measuring spiritual well-being in people with cancer: The functional assessment of chronic illness therapy—spiritual well-being scale (FACIT-sp). *Annals of Behavioral Medicine* 24(1): 49–58.

Puchalski, C. 2002. Spirituality and end-of-life care: A time for listening and caring. *Journal of Palliative Medicine* 5(2): 289–94.

Puchalski, C., et al. 2009. Improving the quality of spiritual care as a dimension of palliative care: The report of the consensus conference. *Journal of Palliative Medicine* 12(10): 885–904.

Pullman, D. 2004. Death, dignity, and moral nonsense. *Journal of Palliative Care* 20(3): 171–77.

Rahner, K. 1971. *Theological investigations VII*. London: Darton, Longman and Todd.

Rose, S. 2001. Is the term 'spirituality' a word that everyone uses, but nobody knows what anyone means by it? *Journal of Contemporary Religion* 16(2): 193–207.

Saunders, C. 2002. Letter to A. Strauss, 19 December 1965. In *Cicely Saunders, founder of the hospice movement: Selected letters 1959–1999*. Oxford: Oxford University Press, 95.

Schwartz, C. E., K. Mazor, J. Rogers, Y. Ma, and G. Reed. 2003. Validation of a new measure of the concept of a good death. *Journal of Palliative Medicine* 6(4): 575–84.

Selman, L., R. Harding, M. Gysels, P. Speck, I. J. Higginson. 2010. The measurement of spirituality in palliative care and the content of tools validated cross-culturally: A systematic review. *Journal of Pain and Symptom Management* 41(4): 728–53.

Shuman, J. J., and K. G. Meador. 2003. *Heal thyself: Spirituality, medicine, and the distortion of Christianity*. Oxford: Oxford University Press.

Sinclair, S. 2011. Impact of death and dying on the personal lives and practices of palliative and hospice care profession-als. *Canadian Medical Association Journal* 183(2): 180–87.

Sinclair, S., M. Mysak, and N. A. Hagen. 2009. What are the core elements of oncology spiritual care programs? *Palliative and Supportive Care* 7: 415–22.

Sinclair, S., J. Pereira, and S. Raffin. 2006a. A thematic review of the spirituality literature within palliative care. *Journal of Palliative Medicine* 9(2): 464–79.

Sinclair, S., S. Raffin, J. Pereira, and N. Guebert. 2006b. Collective soul: The spirituality of an interdisciplinary team. *Palliative and Supportive Care* 4(1): 13–24.

Singer, P. A., D. K. Martin, and M. Kelner. 1999. Quality end-of-life care: Patients' perspectives. *Journal of the American Medical Association* 281: 163–68.

Smith-Stoner, M. 2007. End of life preferences for atheists. *Journal of Palliative Medicine* 10(4): 923–98.

Steinhauser, K. E., N. A. Christakis, E. C. Clipp, M. McNeilly, L. McIntyre, and J. A. Tulsky. 2000. Factors considered important at the end of life by patients, family, physicians, and other care providers. *JAMA* 284(19): 2476–82.

Sullivan, A., K. Hedberg, and D. Fleming. 2000. Legalized physician-assisted suicide in Oregon: The second year. *New England Journal of Medicine* 342(8): 598–604.

Sulmasy, D. 2006. Spiritual issues in the care of dying patients. *JAMA* 296(11): 1385–92.

Tamura, K., K. Ichihara, E. Maetaki, K. Takayama, K. Tanisawa, and M. Ikenaga. 2006. Development of a spiritual pain assessment sheet for terminal cancer patients: Targeting terminal cancer patients admitted to palliative care units in Japan. *Palliative and Supportive Care* 4: 179–88.

Thompson, G., and H. M. Chochinov. 2010. Reducing the potential for suffering in older adults with advanced cancer. *Palliative and Supportive Care* 8: 83–93.

VandeCreek, L., and L. Burton. 2001. Professional chaplaincy: Its role and importance in health care. *Journal of Pastoral Care* 55(1): 81–97.

Vanistendael, S. 2007. Resilience and spirituality. In *Resilience in palliative care*, ed. B. Monroe and D. Oliviere. New York: Oxford, 115–35.

Vivat, B. 2008. Measures of spiritual issues for palliative care patients: A literature review. *Palliative Medicine* 22: 859–68.

Walters, G. 2004. Is there such a thing as a good death? *Palliative Medicine* 18: 404–08.

Webster's international dictionary, 2nd edition. 1946. Springfield, MA: Merriam.

Wilson, K., et al. 2007. Desire for euthanasia or physician-assisted suicide in palliative cancer care. *Health Psychology* 26(3): 314–23.

World Health Organization. 2007. *Definition of palliative care*. Geneva: World Health Organization.

Wright, M. C. 2001. Chaplaincy in hospice and hospital: Findings from a survey in England and Wales. *Palliative Medicine* 15: 229–42.

Zimmermann, C., and G. Rodin. 2004. The denial of death thesis: Sociological critique and implications for palliative care. *Palliative Medicine* 18: 121–28.

CHAPTER 5

Hospice Chaplains, Spirituality, and the Idea of a Good Death

W. WILSON WILL III

Death is also a creative process. We need to be involved. We should not neglect, ignore, or try to solve it. It's an ongoing work of creation.

—A chaplain resident in the United States, 2005

INTRODUCTION

THE PASTORAL CARE of spiritual but not religious (SBNR) patients in hospices presents a set of paradoxes. Chaplains in North America are trained to offer support to individuals of all spiritual traditions and none, yet each is also a leader within a single religion that certifies and supports him or her. They are trained to work with individuals confronting suffering, loss, and uncertainty, yet they may face ambivalence—if not outright hostility—from SBNR individuals wary of religious personnel. Various forms of spiritual expertise, wisdom, and insight held by chaplains may be valued by the SBNR patient, but in the absence of mutual doctrinal foundations, shared cultural outlooks, or even a common spiritual vocabulary, SBNR individuals may wonder if chaplains can understand, much less embrace, their unique spiritual outlooks. Further, to the extent that SBNR persons eschew ecclesiastical hierarchies and favor immediate spiritual experiences, attempts by chaplains

to facilitate spiritual experiences may be awkward at best
and detrimental at worst. Needless to say, lofty pastoral pro-
nouncements or attempts to extract confessions are unlikely to
gain much traction among SBNR persons, for as Chochinov
and Cann suggest, few if any patients are interested in being
"preached" to at life's end (2005, S104). Can hospice chaplains interact therapeutically, humbly, and authentically with
spiritual patients, or will the demands of relativism rob such
encounters of any real substance and leave SBNR individuals to
encounter spiritually impoverished, unsatisfying deaths?

This essay argues that chaplains can indeed help SBNR
persons to make spiritually satisfying use of their time in hospice precisely because these therapeutic spiritual specialists are
skilled at working with spiritually and religiously diverse populations and can utilize this broad knowledge base to support
the personalized beliefs and spiritual practices of SBNR individuals. Spiritual support from such clinical practitioners, firm
in their own spiritual beliefs yet cosmopolitan in their spiritual
outlook, can function as an empathetically compelling resource
for individuals seeking helpful ways to integrate their spiritual
outlook into the hospice journey. Chaplains can offer an unconditional regard for the SBNR individual as a person through
the guarantee of a safe, supportive space in which to explore
spiritual aspects of the mundane and fundamental aspects of
human existence.

This chapter begins with an overview of key conceptual
and practical challenges to the pastoral care of SBNR patients.
Next, it outlines philosophical components of chaplain training
with spiritually diverse populations and provides some examples of the acculturation process of chaplain trainees in clinical
settings regarding hospice as both a philosophy of care and as
a physical place in which this care occurs. Thereafter it ana-
lyzes logistical aspects of pastoral outreach, from establishing
relationships and spiritual assessment to meaning facilitation,
emotional support, and rituals. Final sections discuss pastoral
outreach to family members and friends of patients and to fellow staff members.

Vignettes come primarily from work in a two-year Clinical
Pastoral Education (CPE) training program in a medical center

and hospice in the eastern United States. Residents in the program represent a small, diverse cohort of students from Pentecostal, Baptist, Buddhist, Reformed, Anglican, and Interfaith traditions.

BACKGROUND CONSIDERATIONS

The spiritual roots of hospice care present both challenges and opportunities for chaplains in North America today, as growing interest in spirituality and spiritual diversity meets decreasing denominational affiliation. According to Bradshaw, Cicely Saunders's original vision of hospice care was explicitly Christian and included Protestant chaplains to minister to patients and family members, although clergy and staff members from other religious traditions were also to be welcomed. This openness to religious pluralism reflected Saunders's conviction that patients of all religious traditions and none were welcome and could choose whether or not to utilize the "spiritual help" offered by the chaplain (Bradshaw 1996, 411).

This historical mandate raises two broad sets of questions. First, to what extent is it reasonable or appropriate for religiously affiliated chaplains to offer care to SBNR patients? Second, is it possible—let alone desirable—to maintain fidelity to Saunders's original goals and to help patients to die well in hospices today in light of increasing spiritual diversity?

To answer these questions, it is helpful to consider first the types and stakes of spiritual diversity for various parties involved in hospice pastoral care (for a helpful introduction to broader issues of hospital chaplaincy in North America, see VandeCreek and Burton 2001). First, chaplains often struggle with tensions between their own religious convictions and those of the persons they serve, particularly when there is a large gap between the two. At the same time, the profession as a whole has come under criticism from some quarters regarding openness to spiritual diversity. Engelhardt suggests that the growing professionalization of chaplaincy in recent years has involved a shift "from an identity and goals directed beyond the horizon of the finite" to goals "set within the therapeutic horizon" of biomedicine and its secular, rational outlook. For him, such a shift represents a theological "banalization" of chaplaincy that renders "denominational differences equivalent to aesthetic preferences" (2003, 153). Similar concerns are raised by Delkeskamp-Hayes, who describes such work as "generic" spirituality, "often merely implicit in denominationalist approaches, [which] assumes that some 'absolute' can be prayerfully invoked through the medium of diverse rituals, confessions, and symbols." In her view, this form of spirituality is "meaning-impoverished" and risks blurring the lines between Christianity and "idiosyncratic new age esoteric, updated shamanist, feminism-exploiting witchcrafty, magic arts oriented and benevolent-demon worship" (2003, 8–9).

Several responses come to mind. First, chaplains have long encountered in their clinical work a diversity of personalities, ethnicities, and socioeconomic statuses in ways that have demanded openness to the other and flexibility; such was the case even when patient populations were overwhelmingly Christian. Similarly, there exists enormous diversity of spiritual belief within particular denominations. A liberal Presbyterian chaplain, for example, may hold more in common with an Anglican/Episcopalian, Roman Catholic, Jewish, or even SBNR individual than with a conservative member of her own denomination. A common denominational affiliation is absolutely no guarantee of spiritual consonance in clinical pastoral interactions, making the feasibility of fidelity to a single theological position problematic at best.

That said, some religious leaders are attracted to chaplaincy precisely because the role allows them to work with persons outside their spiritual tradition. Ford, a Buddhist, describes his tradition's openness to multiple spiritual truths as "fluid" in a way that desires all parties in a pastoral relationship to be "nurtured and transformed" by their interactions, particularly when the issue of mortality is at stake (2006, 658). This perspective is all the more important given what he notes as a lack of experience among many individuals applying their spiritual beliefs and convictions to their own finitude. As a caregiver, he argues that "knowing the patient's denomination or general faith background will lend little or no insight into the patient's progress in adapting and applying their deepest beliefs to their situation" (ibid.).

There are also a number of historical reasons for this deliberate openness to spiritual diversity. Lee sees in the evolution of clinical spiritual care in North America a strategic move from a "peripheral service, applicable only to the few 'religious' patients, into an integral element of patient care for all" (2002, 339–40). He explains that psychology and psychoanalysis found a receptive audience in many seminaries and contributed to a new basis for pastoral care, one that placed less emphasis on doctrine and more on relationships and personal insight. Further, he argues that shifts in institutional priorities moved from "clinical pathway-specific applications . . . to more general categories of performance competency" that included such criteria as patient education and rights, organizational ethics, and behavioral health (2002, 341–42), all of which also influenced pastoral care programs. Similar themes are echoed in the popular press, where a "new pastoral model" in health care facilities reflects a shortage of clergy in some denominations, a decline in familiar ritual practices associated with "traditional worship," and shifting beliefs about the efficacy of "spiritual care" among medical professionals (Vitello 2008).

PROFESSIONAL THEOLOGICAL AND ETHICAL STANDARDS

Another key consideration in pastoral relationships near life's end is ethics. Which ethical system ought to be employed when engaging SBNR patients? The patient's? The hospice's? A secular philosophical one? Even if there is agreement that it is desirable for a religious chaplain to meet and support a spiritual patient, it may be far more challenging to discuss actions and behaviors without a shared normative system. Daaleman and VandeCreek argue that religion-based ethics still provides a point of reference for much clinical decision making (2000, 2514), even in secular bioethical standards of nonsectarian hospices and medical centers. In such situations, a chaplain may unconsciously find herself drawing upon her own religious

ethical framework in her spiritual care, yet such a move similarly risks charges of proselytization.

In order to understand how hospice chaplains respond to
these issues, it is helpful to understand a few points about the
training and accreditation processes of health care chaplains in
North America. Key for this chapter is reverent acknowledgment, nonproselytization, and nonjudgment.

Reverent acknowledgment: This core ethos espouses an
unconditional positive regard for all persons as fellow human
beings worthy of compassion, concern, and focused attention.
Reverent acknowledgment emphasizes hospitality toward the
stranger and holds an expansive view of spirituality as a component of the clinical journey that neither privileges one tradition or personal belief system over another nor views a belief
system in the abstract, that is, separate from the way in which
a patient understands it within the context of his or her own
life. This norm is designed to provide a framework for honest,
candid, and confidential exchanges in which one might observe
and cultivate experiences of transcendence and particularly
empowerment among religiously and spiritually diverse populations, including SBNR individuals.

Nonproselytization: Under absolutely no condition is a
chaplain to attempt to convert someone to a new spiritual or
religious tradition (Accreditation Commission 2005). This is a
standard component of pastoral care as specified by the U.S.
Association of Clinical Pastoral Education (ACPE) and the
Canadian Association for Spiritual Care (Association cana-
dienne de soins spirituels; CASC/ACSS). Indeed, it is the duty
of chaplains to "respect the right of each faith group to hold to
its values and traditions" (CASC/ACSS 2009). For some chaplain trainees, this requirement is both intuitive and comfortable; they are equally open to monotheistic, polytheistic, and
atheistic forms of spirituality. Others find this dictate intoler-
able and believe that it violates the very fabric of their religious
commitments, particularly as regards the welfare of a person's
soul as death approaches. For these persons, chaplaincy work is
unlikely to be a viable career option.

Sometimes, however, chaplain trainees find that they are
able to embrace new perspectives regarding evangelization, as

was the case with one Methodist minister at my training site. In her words, "I will always treasure my encounter with the older gentleman who referred to himself as a 'devout atheist' because I was grateful that I was able to respectfully engage him in his hour of need without attempting to convert him, as my early spiritual training had taught me was the goal of personal encounters." Such interactions did not cause this clergywoman to discard her belief in heaven, but they did lead her to rethink her own motivations for connecting with patients.

Nonjudgment: In addition to the prohibition on proselytization, chaplains are trained not to evaluate others' beliefs and actions. Chaplains do not seek to extract confessions or to condemn but to support spiritual healing and growth. True, spiritual care may include conversations about reconciliation with others and may ultimately involve processes of asking and receiving forgiveness, but it is not the place of the chaplain to demand or persuade someone to do these tasks as a prerequisite for acceptance as a person or as a precursor to healing. Such an outlook is extremely important in centers such as HIV/AIDS hospices, where patients may have faced severe stigma and rejection from religious groups and others and yet long to be able to embrace spirituality within their clinical journey. The following anecdote by another chaplain colleague of mine provides additional insights into this ethical duty:

> I remember the young black man who taught me the importance of paying attention to people's faces, which can speak volumes, rather than to the way they are dressed. I approached the young man because there was pain and distress in his countenance. As a result I had a rich encounter with him that would have been missed if I had simply stereotyped him as a young person who probably has no interest in spiritual things.

Here, nonjudgment took the form of providing care to a patient's family member, someone unaccustomed to the culture of the medical space and not religious in any traditional sense yet struggling with profound issues of belief in light of his family member's condition. The lesson for this chaplain was clear:

just as a young adult in "gangster" hip-hop clothing may have profound spiritual yearnings, an elderly gentleman in a cardigan may be far less interested in pondering the meaning of the cosmos or discussing his sense of the supernatural than in watching the golf tournament on TV.

Beyond these professional norms, chaplains navigate the formal ethical regulations of the hospices in which they work, the religious ethical mandates of their own religious tradition, and the spiritual ethical leanings of SBNR patients. While a more thorough discussion of this topic is beyond the scope of this chapter, two points deserve mention here. First, the regulations of Canadian armed forces chaplains present a basic formula that applies for hospices as well: "minister to our own—care for all—facilitate worship of others" (Ministry of National Defence 2005, iv). Second, recent writings in cross-cultural bioethics may also prove helpful as chaplains and other clinicians wrestle with principlist- versus casuist-based reasoning in their work with SBNR patients and others whose traditions do not neatly align with a single Western religious or philosophical tradition (see, e.g., Turner 2004).

ESTABLISHING PASTORAL RELATIONSHIPS

Given these ethical considerations, how are chaplains trained to behave in their initial meetings with SBNR patients? This segment discusses contact between the patient and the hospice both prior to and following admission.

Before hospice: Frequently, a social worker establishes contact with a patient contemplating hospice care and inquires about the person's spiritual needs and preferences (Hall 1997, 221). Such information can be extremely useful for understanding the basics of a person's spirituality, thoughts about his or her physical body and medical condition, beliefs about death, and social and relational priorities. In this respect, it is arguably just as important to make sure that chaplains are available for consultation as such choices are weighed; such work could include coordination with a chaplain at the patient's hospital prior to the move to hospice, in order to promote continuity of spiritual care and to note any special preferences or concerns. In cases of limited pastoral resources, admissions personnel can at least ensure the presence of an SBNR option on intake forms for the benefit of those who will care for the patient.

In hospice: How do chaplains get in contact with patients after admission? Policies vary from institution to institution but typically include patient requests, referrals from staff or family members, and rounds by the chaplain on a unit. Importantly, though, they should be consistent and, in the case of staff referrals, should be made "in the same manner" as referrals to other clinical specialists regarding disclosure of intentions to the patient (LaRocca-Pitts 2008, 4).

That said, in the same way that it is important to understand a prospective patient's views on the relationship between spirituality and hospice care, it is vital to obtain an accurate sense of a person's impressions of chaplains as early as possible in a patient's stay, particularly given Cairns's reminder about the enormous destructive potential of spirituality and religion (1999, 452). Harvey finds that clinical chaplains may be perceived as everything from shamans and miracle workers to arbiters, telephone operators, social workers, and friends (1996, 42). Special sensitivity is appropriate during all initial interactions between chaplains and others in the hospice environment, for while the very presence of a hospice chaplain is unlikely to raise the specter of death in ways that it may in a general hospital, the introduction of a chaplain into the dying process of SBNR individuals may arouse concern, suspicion, or even hostility, particularly if the initial meeting results from a staff referral.

Several practical measures can be taken to help address these concerns, including written information on spiritual resources available in the hospice and introductions by admissions or other staff members. When a chaplain knows of or senses apprehension during this first meeting, he or she may wish to explain the nature of his or her role with a spiritually diverse patient population (especially with respect to the professional standards outlined earlier). Chochinov and Cann suggest that end-of-life spirituality should be a highly egalitarian process that minimizes paternalism and hierarchies in favor of a partnership model (2005, S106). SBNR patients may not be accustomed to working with any professional on such topics, so a chaplain can provide reassurance by letting them know that their spiritual convictions and inklings are welcome in the hospice. A former colleague explained the evolution of her thinking about initial meetings in the following way:

> As far as the appropriate use of spiritual/religious resources is concerned, I now allow the one I am encountering to choose between me praying *for* them or *with* them, which some seem to find refreshing. I let them know that although I am the chaplain I am not "pushing prayers." I realize that there are a huge number of people that do not have an active life of faith and although they may want prayer, some may feel uncomfortable or even sacrilegious participating in a prayer. [Emphasis in original]

This chaplain realized that even a few words of clarification could reassure patients with spiritual yearnings unaccustomed to participating in formal religious rituals such as prayer and thus found herself increasingly comfortable working with a broader range of patients and spiritualities.

SPIRITUAL SCREENINGS, HISTORIES, AND ASSESSMENTS

Beyond initial introductions, the question of how chaplains and SBNR patients can make good use of finite time together remains. This section focuses on mechanisms that help to understand a hospice patient's spiritual state and to discern which spiritual resources from chaplains will be most beneficial.

What does it mean "to die appropriately" (Hermann 2001, 68)? How can chaplains work with SBNR patients toward this goal? Several different types of clinical spiritual activities merit consideration here. Derrickson separates spiritual support from spiritual intervention (1996, 13), where the former emphasizes a more passive, nurturing role for the chaplain and the latter a more active, therapeutic, or ameliorative set of tasks. Fitchett, meanwhile, distinguishes between spiritual screening and spiritual assessment, where the former is akin to triage and the latter a more extensive process designed "to determine whether or not a patient has spiritual risk and to provide the information needed to shape the spiritual care that will address the spiritual risk" (1999, 8–9).

Nonetheless, as previous chapters in this book demonstrate, many definitions of spirituality exist, and each of these definitions contains values and priorities that may be relevant to an SBNR person's current state of spiritual health and understanding of a good death. Such diversity can make screenings and assessments of SBNR patients by chaplains less straightforward than assessments of denominationally affiliated patients.

One way for a chaplain and the SBNR patient to begin these processes is to discuss the latter's sense of connection between his spiritual beliefs and his health (see Johnson 2001, 184). In particular, does he or she maintain that there exists a relationship between bodily death and the continuation of some sort of consciousness, self, or soul after physical demise? Some SBNR individuals may have undergone several shifts in belief or perspective in years prior to hospice admission and so may not have a tidy sense of spiritual identity, set of spiritual resources, or clear convictions regarding end-of-life spirituality (see Lim et al. 2010). For these persons, it may be helpful to discuss the patient's sense of hospice as a continuation or break from previous spiritual experiences. What are the patient's hopes and expectations from hospice as far as spiritual development is concerned? Does he or she have a vision of how he or she would like to incorporate spirituality into the dying process? Indeed, a patient may have well-worn methods for engaging the spiritual that may or may not include other persons, or that individual may be struggling with new sentiments and may seek insights on how to proceed.

A few words of caution are needed at this point. Newer chaplains may be unconsciously inclined to view disease, suffering, and death from the perspectives of (their own) religious viewpoints and previous life experiences and may structure initial diagnostic questions accordingly. An awareness of the sorts

of priorities and biases that these individuals possess regarding
fears of death and the unknown is valuable for their professional ability and willingness to accompany an SBNR patient
on such a journey. The following reflections from a Presbyterian minister from Africa training in a large U.S. care facility
exemplify some of these struggles:

> I . . . appreciate my encounter with the partner of a man
> with AIDS-related pneumonia. I found myself truly
> grateful that I have matured to the point of ministering
> without being judgmental. I was able to honor this indi-
> vidual as a person in pain and anguish over the health
> of his loved one. He mentioned some of the difficulties
> they had encountered in the church, but I did not make
> that the centerpiece of my ministry to him, as would
> have been the case before I had ever taken a CPE unit.

SBNR individuals may be reluctant to discuss spiritual beliefs
with chaplains, particularly if the former perceive that the latter hold religious views about life after death that deemphasize
thoughts about the present in favor of some future existence
defined by a religious tradition (Cicirelli 2011, 130). Indeed,
a person who selects hospice care may not believe in life after
death and hence may wish to live this life as long as possible
while simply rejecting further biomedical intervention (141).
In such a situation, the chaplain may wish to focus on topics
of life satisfaction, gaining meaning from life in its beauty and
fullness, helping to foster congruence between hospice lifestyle
and spiritual beliefs, and nurturing a sense of community and
connection within the hospice. Likewise, the chaplain may wish
to invite patients to find ways to support each other or teach
others about dying (Daaleman and VandeCreek 2000, 2515).
    Furthermore, chaplains are trained to be attentive to signs
of spiritual suffering; they watch for factors that may inhibit
an SBNR patient's ability to draw upon spirituality helpfully to
attain the sort of good death that patient desires. Such factors
can include physical or psychological problems or other non-
verbal manifestations, including feelings of hopelessness and
worthlessness as well as a sense of meaninglessness. Spiritual

suffering may likewise exacerbate, and be exacerbated by, physical pain and may potentially complicate diagnostic and therapeutic strategies (Rousseau 2000, 2000–01), both spiritual and
psychological.

When there is evidence of spiritual suffering, chaplains may
wish to ask about a patient's spiritual coping methods to see
if these resources can contribute to the desired positive results
or if they instead parallel "negative religious coping" methods
that can be indicative of distress and impaired quality of life
(Hills et al. 2005, 782). More research is needed on the concept
of negative spiritual coping, but it is important for chaplains to
be open to this possibility, in the same way that they learn to
distinguish between spiritual issues, spiritual distress, and spiritual crises for SBNR individuals in the hospice setting (Derrickson 1996, 17).

Similarly, a variety of demographic factors may influence
spiritual diagnostic processes; some SBNR individuals will be
more inclined to reveal aspects of their lives to chaplains than
others, and these factors may complicate attempts to understand a patient's spiritual state. Gender may play a significant
role in determining the use of spiritual resources and in openness to verbalizing inner thoughts and feelings with others.
Hermann, for example, argues that women may report more
"unmet spiritual needs" than men (2001, 75), while Logan et
al. suggest that women may desire "focused isolation" in which
to reflect without interacting with a chaplain or other spiritual
care providers (2006, 121), and Chandler concludes that while
men "may not have had the inclination" to pursue such matters, many women "have not had the time" to do so (1999, 70).
Similarly, generational differences may lead to variation in concepts of need and openness to discussion of patients' personal
lives with a religious figure. More research is needed to validate such claims, yet these preliminary findings are nonetheless
valuable to the extent that they introduce questions about the
extent of social influences on spiritual expression in the hospice
environment.

Additional factors may be considered as part of a chaplain's
spiritual assessment of an SBNR patient. These include concerns about forgiveness and alienated relationships; desire to

be in the presence of a benevolent higher power; sense of connection to the natural environment (Puchalski 2002, 290); the nature of the social world from which a patient is moving into hospice; and ruptures or continuities with regard to issues of safety, predictability, and connection with loved ones. Also, the spiritual needs of patients and their families may vary between pediatric and adult hospices; this too is a topic in need of further research.

Finally, it is important to note that at least in the United States, there are a number of highly pragmatic, institutional rationales that impinge upon spiritual diagnostic activities, above and beyond the obvious concerns for the welfare of patients and others. Lee argues that through the use of "spiritual assessment," chaplains consider the "whole person" to document specific sites of intervention and to justify their work to hospital administrators (2002, 344). For him, pastoral assessment also fits productively with the rise of "patient empowerment and medical consumerism . . . without challenging the centrality of the biomedical perspective" (2002, 346). Similarly, spiritual assessment of SBNR individuals in the United States can be invaluable yet may prove challenging in terms of federal hospice regulations, especially due to the categorical nature of many religious/spiritual scales that encourages routinization and, according to Garces-Foley, discourages the sort of spontaneous and sensitive care required by SBNR persons (2006, 125). Given such regulations, it may be appropriate to assess patients' changing spiritual experiences, needs, and abilities over time (Chochinov and Cann 2005, S103) and have the chaplain document and monitor these issues on behalf of the care team.

DISCOURSE, INTERPRETATION, AND MEANING

As previously suggested, the structure and content of diagnostic pastoral conversations is a central component of interactions between hospice chaplains and SBNR patients. Supportive pastoral communication can likewise take a variety of spoken and unspoken forms that include life review, readings from sacred texts, body language, and silence, yet differences of opinion exist regarding the therapeutic value of talking near life's end. Bradshaw questions this linguistic turn in hospice chaplaincy, arguing that in the United Kingdom, at least, "traditional values meant the showing of love often in silence and quiet whereas modern approaches presume verbal activity, counseling, talking, self-expression; [and] 'getting in touch with feelings' by expressing them" (1996, 414). Conversely, Dobratz's study of the relationship between pain and expressed spirituality in a home hospice population in the United States suggests that for at least some individuals, there is a positive correlation between self-reported pain and nonexpressed spirituality (2005, 243), a finding that warrants investigation with regard to chaplains and SBNR patients.

Whatever the amount of verbal exchange, meaning and spirituality are intimately related to the use of language in hospice care. Meaning is mentioned routinely in discussions about medical care, suffering, and healing, yet its clinical relevance is typically unarticulated. At a most basic level, meaning is a linguistic practice of ascribing significance to objects and events. From my own experience working in hospice and other clinical environments, the desire for meaning in light of a particular event connotes a search for relevance, for either a person's identity or worldview. Medical events, in other words, do not simply happen; they imply something. Particularly for SBNR patients, attempts may be made to set bodily events within a framework of meaning, purpose, and dignity.

With their expertise in nonjudgmental listening and interpretation, chaplains are well suited to working with SBNR individuals to help interpret thoughts and images that arise in the hospice space, especially as patients seek insight against the backdrop of regnant social norms and modes of viewing death. Similarly, chaplains can help patients to find a (greater) sense of control over life. Indeed, individuals may experience some spiritual growth in hospices but may also encounter "dissonance" if facility with spiritual thoughts and resources is elementary or is at odds with the person's life up to that point (Hinshaw 2005, 264–65). Here in particular, chaplains can reassure SBNR patients that the search for spiritual meaning can be tentative and unorthodox; they can remind them that ambiguous or fluid beliefs are legitimate and do not reflect deficiency on the part of their spirituality or their beliefs. For example, one pediatrics chaplain at my site realized that interpretative encouragement held important implications for her patients and for their ability to connect with the transcendent. "My philosophy of pastoral care is very cautious in ensuring that the provider is not imposing his or her own ideas of what the communication between the recipient and God should be. This is most simply achieved by a rigorous adherence to the discipline of reverent acknowledgement." She found this perspective particularly important working on oncology, where children's understandings of the divine were often unconventional by traditional religious standards yet breathtakingly profound in their sincerity and insight.

Similarly, hospice chaplains may be asked to help interpret signs from patients and family members wrestling with profound existential concerns yet whose spiritual beliefs may not provide immediately obvious solutions to their thoughts or experiences. Such challenges can result in interpretative scenarios in which sensitive creativity may be required in order to bring about a measure of cohesion to the person's worldview. Chaplains can thus help SBNR individuals to distinguish the "implicit meaning" of medical information from "found meaning" (Daaleman and VandeCreek 2000, 2515), a more active, creative process in which a person works to find insight and place such information within broader cognitive, emotional, and spiritual contexts.

Regarding the logistics of pastoral meetings, chaplains can help to facilitate a suitable clinical environment appropriate for patients to reflect individually on their search for meaning. This may include routine rest hours, a chapel or "reading/quiet room facilities" for mobile patients, and screens for others. For those whose spirituality is connected to a community of others, larger spaces such as a dining hall may be appropriate (Johnson 2001, 179).

ADDITIONAL INTERVENTIONS WITH
PATIENTS AND WITH FAMILY MEMBERS

Pastoral outreach to SBNR hospice patients can take additional forms that are both related to and distinct from language.

Chaplains cannot literally die with their patients, but they can be loyal companions for a significant portion of the hospice journey (Burns 1991, 48). They are well positioned to offer "a presence of security and peace in a world" that may seem "to be crumbling down" (Hall 1997, 221). For example, through their pledge of confidentiality, chaplains can provide patients the opportunity to share concerns that they might not otherwise reveal to others. Chaplains also discuss a variety of items related to patient care with fellow staff members and with friends and family of SBNR patients, and insights gleaned from these various parties can help to give chaplains a uniquely insightful understanding of the various meanings and concerns that these multiple actors bring to a case. A deeply mystical interfaith chaplain colleague summarized this aspect of her work with reference to transcendent beings:

> Another common angelic role is that of guardian angel or protector. In my philosophy of pastoral care, I interpret this as a reference to the possibility for the pastoral care provider to act as an advocate for those they serve. We are in a unique position to be an intermediary or even a champion of our patients and families if necessary.

The capacity of the chaplain to function as neutral party or mediator can play a significant role in an SBNR patient's relationships in hospice. They can do so by identifying points of common ground between parties, clarifying misunderstandings, working to foster reconciliation when possible, ensuring that an SBNR patient's last wishes are respected, and intervening if someone attempts to hijack her spiritual journey or otherwise challenges her dignity.

Returning briefly to the topic of ethics, cross-cultural communication and non-Western bioethical norms regarding the rights and duties of the patient can raise significant challenges in hospice care (Crawley et al. 2002, 674). While such issues may not directly fall under the rubric of spirituality, disagreements about decision making and competing priorities about topics such as sacraments or other rituals can impact hospice spiritual journeys when an SBNR patient's beliefs diverge from those of family members. In such situations, it may be particularly challenging for chaplains to coordinate care in light of overlapping role perceptions or customs that do not align neatly with the patient's own spiritual framework. Chaplains working in ethnically diverse urban areas in particular may find it advantageous to become familiar with the spiritual and religious priorities of local cultural groups to help caregivers and others at the hospice to appreciate the nuances of diverse end-of-life traditions and values as they impinge upon the beliefs of SBNR patients. In more challenging cases in which family members demand certain religious rituals or activities that the SBNR individual rejects, chaplains may find themselves defending the patient's autonomy and ultimately denying family members or others their wishes. Such conundrums may be painful for all involved yet are acute possibilities for SBNR patients, and it is thus important for chaplains—and hospices more generally—to talk frankly about their willingness to take such steps on behalf of SBNR patients, even at the risk of alienating a patient's religious family members and friends. Such disputes may be particularly complicated in pediatric hospices and warrant further research.

At the same time, while patients are the chief concern of hospice chaplains, they are by no means the only ones whom they seek to support in the clinical setting. Chaplains are particularly well suited to supporting family members and friends throughout the hospice experience, whether or not there is spiritual tension between an SBNR patient and visitors. The chaplain can listen sincerely to their concerns and reflections, propose channels for communication, and explain the cultural values and priorities of SBNR patients to other staff members. Chaplains can also help family members to process their own religious, spiritual, and emotional thoughts as their relative undertakes the hospice journey. They can offer education, for instance by sharing insights about what other patients have described, or experienced, in part to help familiarize the patient to the myriad of thoughts and sensations that may occur. As Harvey suggests, chaplains can present themselves as students, eager to listen as an individual shares his or her insights and reminisces over years past. They can also offer suggestions on topics such as coping, learning new ways of relating to the self and others, and forgiveness and reconciliation (1996, 43).

SPIRITUALITY AND FELLOW STAFF MEMBERS

Turning now to spiritual care and the relationship between chaplains and other hospice staff members, a key consideration is the uniqueness (or exclusivity) of spiritual care of SBNR patients by chaplains. Few would dispute the appropriateness of an ordained priest's administering a sacrament to a patient belonging to that denomination, but is a chaplain the only person qualified to broach spirituality with SBNR individuals? Could this work be performed as well—if not better—by other members of a hospice care team, particularly by colleagues who have not been steeped in organized religion? In some cases, I believe the answer is yes. Previous essays in this volume have discussed the challenges and opportunities faced by nurses, social workers, and others and will not be rehearsed here. Nonetheless, a few remarks are in order.

Increasingly, it appears that many individual hospice clinicians want to engage patients on a spiritual level as part of their duties—or believe that they are already doing so (Harding et al. 2008, 101, 112). While such desires may be extremely selfless and heartfelt, motivation of course does not guarantee competence. As Handzo and Koenig intimate, it is one thing for a clinician to conduct a brief spiritual screening as a spiritual "generalist" and quite another to attempt to interact with a patient as a "specialist" (2004, 1242). This is particularly the case with SBNR patients, whose beliefs and practices are unlikely to present a familiar or coherent schema to clinicians not explicitly trained to work with them (see Johnson 2001, 181–82). Chaplains may wish to work with staff members conducting spiritual screenings to ensure that they are appropriate for SBNR individuals. Similarly, chaplains may wish to highlight the fact that (recent statistical analyses of topics such as intercessory prayer notwithstanding) notions of efficacy in spiritual care are conceptualized somewhat differently than in other aspects of clinical practice. A lack of clearly identifiable, quantifiable data on spiritual outcomes should not undermine confidence in a person's potential to contribute to an SBNR hospice patient's spiritual journey (see Kristeller et al. 1999, 451).

Nonetheless, the reality of anticlericalism within several cohorts in our society is such that the mere presence of a chaplain may breed wariness or even hostility among some SBNR individuals in hospices. In these cases, a thoughtfully equipped nurse, physician, social worker, or even janitor may in fact be in the best position to engage and assuage such a person, especially if she has developed a positive rapport with the patient and feels comfortable communicating with him about spiritual issues. To this end, a pastoral care department may wish to offer workshops to colleagues on topics such as nonjudgmental listening, guided meditation, and family dynamics in order to provide basic training for staff members who wish to receive such training.

Conversely, just as some SBNR individuals may be wary of chaplains, it is possible that some religious staff members may take exception to what they see as heterodox, vague, or wishy-washy beliefs and outlooks among SBNR patients and may chafe at the idea of seemingly pagan or heathen rituals or practices occurring in the hospice environment. Chaplains are well positioned to help fellow staff members to process their own thoughts about spiritual diversity among the dying and to discuss anxieties that they may have about the fate of those whose spiritual beliefs differ from their own.

Even if there is no tension regarding SBNR beliefs or chaplains present, the notion of spiritual dimensions of care (Chochinov and Cann 2005, S105) is both plausible and compelling, and for those staff members so inclined, chaplains can help them to think consciously about aspects of their own work as spiritually nurturing activities. Moreover, given evidence that hospice spiritual care is increasingly conducted apart from—or even in the absence of—staff chaplains (Garces-Foley 2006, 130) or chaplain volunteers (Williams et al. 2004, 643), such alternative forms of spiritual support may become more widespread in the future. Assuaging pain, listening, and other palliative interventions can indeed be conducted by other clinicians with sympathy for spirituality, even if such a mindset is not stated explicitly. So long as the collective outreach of the care team is consistent in its spiritual messages and aims, patients who desire such support can only stand to benefit from such widespread compassion. At centers in which a chaplain is not routinely present, administrators may wish to consider inviting a suitably trained chaplain to conduct occasional workshops for staff members on care for SBNR patients. Suitable topics might include definitions of spirituality and religion, special issues commonly faced by SBNR patients at the end of life, spiritual distress, diversity among how SBNR patients view and address death and dying (see Marr et al. 2007, 170), and knowing how to distinguish psychosocial constructs of illness and death from spiritual ones (Daaleman and VandeCreek 2000, 2515).

Finally, multiple members of a care team and even friends and family (Lunn 2003, 161) may be able to contribute uniquely and positively to the spiritual care of SBNR patients. So long as this work is coordinated, for instance through a mechanism such as spirituality rounds, the outcome may be positive for all involved (Clark et al. 2007, 1321).

CONCLUSION

In a sense, the ideal hospice chaplain is the spiritual equivalent of an ethnobotanist: someone familiar with the tools and taxonomies of a wide range of spiritual systems and movements, from the structured to the eclectic, who can appreciate the beliefs and practices that SBNR patients and others hold. Such mastery represents a large investment that may not be feasible or even practical in areas with relatively homogenous patient populations. Still, as demographic trends shift in North America, hospices will do well to consider the multicultural and multispiritual expertise of employees and may wish to think carefully about how chaplains may be able to help facilitate such components of care as part of their work with SBNR persons.

While the diversity presented by spiritual but not religious patients in hospices could be viewed as a cause for concern for more denominationally oriented chaplains, I suggest that the presence of such patients near life's end can offer important opportunities to reconsider the very concept of chaplaincy in terms of function and identity. Further, the evolution—if that is the right word for it—of patient populations need not imply that pastoral care is redundant but can, in fact, be seen as the fulfillment of religious duties and can simultaneously honor Saunders's original vision of hospice care.

REFERENCES

Accreditation Commission. 2005. Accreditation manual 2005. Decatur, GA: Association for Clinical Pastoral Education, Inc.

Bradshaw, A. 1996. The spiritual dimension of hospice: The secularization of an ideal. Social Science & Medicine 43(3): 409–19.

Burns, S. 1991. The spirituality of dying: Pastoral care's holistic approach is crucial in hospice. Health Progress 72(7): 48–52, 54.

Cairns, A. B. 1999. Spirituality and religiosity in palliative care. Home Health Care Nurse 17(7): 450–55.

CASC/ACSS. 2009. CAPPE/ACPEP Code of ethics for chaplains, pastoral counselors, pastors, pastoral educators and students. In Handbook. Ingramport, NS: CASC/ACSS.

Chandler, E. 1999. Spirituality. The Hospice Journal 14(3-4): 63–74.

Chochinov, H. M., and B. J. Cann. 2005. Interventions to enhance the spiritual aspects of dying. Journal of Palliative Medicine 8 Suppl. 1: S103–S115.

Cicirelli, V. G. 2011. Religious and nonreligious spirituality in relation to death acceptance or rejection. Death Studies 35(2): 124.

Clark, L., S. Leedy, L. McDonald, B. Muller, C. Lamb, T. Mendez, S. Kim, and R. Schonwetter. 2007. Spirituality and job satisfaction among hospice interdisciplinary team members. Journal of Palliative Medicine 10(6): 1321–28.

Crawley, L. M., P. A. Marshall, B. Lo, and B. A. Koenig, for the End-of-Life Care Consensus Panel. 2002. Strategies for culturally effective end-of-life care. *Annals of Internal Medicine* 136(9): 673–79.

Daaleman, T. P., and L. VandeCreek. 2000. Placing religion and spirituality in end-of-life care. *JAMA: The Journal of the American Medical Association* 284(19): 2514–17.

Delkeskamp-Hayes, C. 2003. Generic versus Catholic hospital chaplaincy: The diversity of spirits as a problem of interfaith cooperation. *Christian Bioethics* 9(1): 3–21.

Derrickson, B. S. 1996. The spiritual work of the dying: A framework and case studies. *The Hospice Journal* 11(2): 11–30.

Dobratz, M. C. 2005. A comparative study of life-closing spirituality in home hospice patients. *Research and Theory for Nursing Practice* 19(3): 243–56.

Engelhardt, H. T., Jr. 2003. The dechristianization of Christian hospital chaplaincy: Some bioethics reflections on professionalization, ecumenization, and secularization. *Christian Bioethics* 9(1): 139–60.

Fitchett, G. 1999. Screening for spiritual risk. *Chaplaincy Today* 15(1): 2–12.

Ford, T. 2006. Interacting with patients of a different faith: The personal reflection of a Buddhist chaplain. *Southern Medical Journal* 99(6): 658–59.

Garces-Foley, K. 2006. Hospice and the politics of spirituality. *Omega* 53(1-2): 117–36.

Hall, S. E. 1997. Spiritual diversity: A challenge for hospice chaplains. *American Journal of Hospice & Palliative Care* 14(5): 221–23.

Handzo, G., and H. G. Koenig. 2004. Spiritual care: Whose job is it anyway? *Southern Medical Journal* 97(12): 1242–44.

Harding, S. R., K. J. Flannelly, K. Galek, and H. P. Tannenbaum. 2008. Spiritual care, pastoral care, and chaplains: Trends in the health care literature. *Journal of Health Care Chaplaincy* 14(2): 99–117.

Harvey, T. 1996. Who is the chaplain anyway? Philosophy and integration of hospice chaplaincy. *American Journal of Hospice and Palliative Medicine* 13(5): 41–43.

Hermann, C. P. 2001. Spiritual needs of dying patients: A qualitative study. *Oncology Nursing Forum* 28(1): 67–72.

Hills, J., J. A. Paice, J. R. Cameron, and S. Shott. 2005. Spirituality and distress in palliative care consultation. *Journal of Palliative Medicine* 8(4): 782–88.

Hinshaw, D. B. 2005. Spiritual issues in surgical palliative care. *Surgical Clinics of North America* 85(2): 257–72.

Johnson, C. P. 2001. Assessment tools: Are they an effective approach to implementing spiritual health care within the NHS? *Accident and Emergency Nursing* 9(3): 177–86.

Kristeller, J. L., C. S. Zumbrun, and R. F. Schilling. 1999. "I would if I could": How oncologists and oncology nurses address spiritual distress in cancer patients. *Psycho-Oncology* 8(5): 451–58.

LaRocca-Pitts, M. A. 2008. FACT: Taking a spiritual history in a clinical setting. *Journal of Health Care Chaplaincy* 15(1): 1–12.

Lee, S. J. C. 2002. In a secular spirit: Strategies of clinical pastoral education. *Health Care Analysis: HCA: Journal of Health Philosophy and Policy* 10(4): 339–56.

Lim, C., C. A. MacGregor, and R. Putnam. 2010. Secular and liminal: Discovering heterogeneity among religious nones. *Journal for the Scientific Study of Religion* 49(4): 596–618.

Logan, J., R. Hackbusch-Pinto, and C. E. De Grasse. 2006. Women undergoing breast diagnostics: The lived experience of spirituality. *Oncology Nursing Forum* 33(1): 121–26.

Lunn, J. S. 2003. Spiritual care in a multi-religious context. *Journal of Pain and Palliative Care Pharmacotherapy* 17(3-4): 153–166; discussion 167–69.

Marr, L., J. A. Billings, and D. E. Weissman. 2007. Spirituality training for palliative care fellows. *Journal of Palliative Medicine* 10(1): 169–77.

Ministry of National Defence, Land Force. 2005. *The chaplain's manual*. Ottawa: Government of Canada.

Puchalski, C. M. 2002. Spirituality and end-of-life care: A time for listening and caring. *Journal of Palliative Medicine* 5(2): 289–94.

Rousseau, P. 2000. Spirituality and the dying patient. *Journal of Clinical Oncology* 18(9): 2000–02.

Turner, L. 2004. Bioethics in pluralistic societies. *Medicine, Health Care and Philosophy* 7(2): 201–08.

VandeCreek, L., and L. Burton, eds. 2001. Professional chaplaincy: Its role and importance in health care. *Journal of Pastoral Care* 55(1): 81–97.

Vitello, P. 2008. Hospice chaplains take up bedside counseling. *New York Times*, October 29, sec. New York Region.

Williams, M. L., M. Wright, M. Cobb, and C. Shiels. 2004. A prospective study of the roles, responsibilities and stresses of chaplains working within a hospice. *Palliative Medicine* 18(7): 638–45.

CHAPTER 6

Tragedy and the Eternal Yea

A Personal Reflection on Atheism

PATRICK GRANT

THE PRESENCE OF AN ABSENCE

IN JUNE 2010, a teleconference took place during which the contributors to the present book introduced themselves to one another and discussed what the project should try to achieve. Three of us could not attend, but we all received a printed summary of the proceedings. Among other things, the participants described their backgrounds and credentials, and these were duly noted in the summary—with one exception. One participant, that is, failed to be listed among those having credentials relevant to "the area of research" in question. It won't be hard for you to guess who.

I begin in this mildly unpromising way because, perhaps counterintuitively, I found the (no doubt accidental) elision surprisingly relieving and, even, unexpectedly relevant. The relief comes from the fact that I am not able to offer "new knowledge to scholars and students of health care and religious studies" as the project requires, and I cannot with any credibility deal with case studies or "narrative clinical examples." Consequently, I find myself constrained to proceed by an alternative route. I even feel quietly encouraged to do so by reason of the aforementioned elision, which I now interpret as slyly supportive of the license I want to take.

The unexpected relevance that I have mentioned arises from the fact that, as it happens, omissions, elisions, and aporias are central to what I want to say in the following pages, both about atheism and also about communicating effectively with terminally ill people. To explain what I mean by this, I would like to begin, not with a case study, but by citing two poems. I limit myself to the three final stanzas of each, on the grounds that these will suffice for our purposes. Also, I label the poems 1 and 2, omitting the authors' names in order to highlight the main question I want to ask about them. Here they are, poems 1 and 2:

1.

But is there for the night a resting place?
   A roof for when the slow dark hours begin.
May not the darkness hide it from my face?
   You cannot miss that inn.

Shall I meet other wayfarers at night?
   Those who have gone before.
Then must I knock, or call when just in sight?
   They will not keep you standing at that door.

Shall I find comfort, travel-sore and weak?
   Of labour you shall find the sum.
Will there be beds for me and all who seek?
   Yea, beds for all who come.

2.

And if as a lad grows older
   The troubles he bears are more,
He carries his griefs on a shoulder
   That handselled them long before.
Where shall one halt to deliver
   This luggage I'd lief set down?
Not Thames, not Teme is the river,
   Nor London nor Knighton the town:

'Tis a long way further than Knighton,
  A quieter place than Clun,
Where doomsday may thunder and lighten
  And little 'twill matter to one.

Both of these sets of verses are about the end of life. The first is a dialogue between someone on a journey and an unidentified respondent. The pilgrim (let us say) asks the questions, and an authoritative voice responds. The second is also about a journey. Here we are addressed by a single speaker, and the only dialogical moment occurs in the second stanza, where the speaker asks a question and then answers it.

In broad terms, both poems tell us the same thing: at the end of life lies the grave, the one fact we can be sure of. It takes a moment to realize that this is what the dead-certain voice in poem 1 is telling the pilgrim, who seems to hope for something more consoling. Will there be a resting place, other wayfarers, comfort? Yes, says the dead-certain respondent, there will be "beds for all who come," and even in the dark you can't miss the "inn," because everybody who has gone before will have a bed there. In short, the grave lies at the end, as inevitable and stark as the replies that, interestingly, allow the pilgrim to keep hoping while nonetheless declaring the bleak truth unflinchingly. It's a chilling little poem, and there is more to say about it, but let's move on to poem 2.

Poem 2 is also about the grave, the one sure thing. The young man has been traveling, and now that he is older, he wonders where and how he can set down his baggage. In the earlier stanzas, he had looked for quiet places in England, and now he repeats the familiar, comforting names, none more quiet than soft-sounding rural Clun. And yet, there is a quieter place even still, and when you get there—as you surely will—the rest of your search won't matter. Not even the trump of doom will disturb you then.

There are various ways to describe the differences between these poems—differences that express a personal signature conveyed through tone, imagery, and the deployment of rhyme and meter. But these differences do not alter the central point: both poems are about what lies at the end of life's journey, and both say, the grave—nothing more.

Now to my question. One of these poems was written by a devout Christian, and the other by a strenuous atheist. Which is which, and what are your reasons for choosing?

As a moment's reflection shows, the answer to this question is not obvious, and if you do get the answer right, too much certainty about the self-evidence of your choice would be, I suggest, suspect. This is so because both poems could feasibly be written either by a believer or an unbeliever, and in both cases the poetry outreaches the descriptive terms "atheist" and "Christian," even though these terms accurately describe certain core convictions of our two authors (the first of whom, by the way, is Christina Rosetti the ardent Christian; the second is A. E. Housman the flinty atheist).[1] Nor is it merely the case, as I might seem to suggest, that the poetry is complex and the labels simple. When we consider the terms "atheist" and "Christian" more closely, they in turn open up upon complexities, so that the opposition between them can easily become unclear.

"ATHEIST," "AGNOSTIC": WHAT THE WORDS (DON'T) TELL US

Early Christians, for instance, were denounced and abominated as atheists, as the second-century Christian apologist Tatian the Syrian tells us (Ryland 1994, 27). Tatian's teacher, Justin Martyr, went a step further in denouncing the execution of Socrates, who was also charged with atheism. Justin saw an affinity between Socrates and the second-century Christians who were likewise accused, and in making this suggestion, Justin stands at the beginning of a Christian humanism that would argue that the pagan Greeks had true insight into the divine logos.

The main reason for early Christians being accused of atheism is that the Romans thought the Christian God unacceptably different from what the Emperor cult required. Yet, surprisingly, from within Christianity itself during the Middle Ages, the most advanced mystics could come perilously close both to atheism and heresy. Meister Eckhart (1260–1327) is a favorite repository of examples of this kind of thing. When at death we go back into the depths, he tells us, "no one will ask," and "God passes away" as we "sink down eternally from nothingness to nothingness" (Sermons and Collations, LVI, XCIX). What does it mean to say that God passes away and at the end there is only nothingness?

In the twentieth century, the respected theologian Paul Tillich is no less provocative when he comments on an argument by Thomas Aquinas about the identity of God's essence and existence. Tillich wants to push Aquinas further, and in so doing concludes that "to argue that God exists is to deny him" (Tillich 1973, 205). Many (perhaps most) Christians would feel uneasy about that. No wonder that David Hume (1711–1776), the Enlightenment philosopher who remains the darling of philosophically minded atheists, saw a close affinity between atheism and mysticism. In *Dialogues Concerning Natural Religion* (Hume 1779), one of the participants, Cleanthes, makes the point:

> those who maintain the perfect simplicity of the Supreme Being, to the extent in which you have explained it, are complete mystics, and chargeable with the consequences which I have drawn from their opinion. They are, in a word, ATHEISTS, without knowing it. (63)

Admittedly, a suitably adjusted historical understanding can rescue the provocative statements of the Christian mystics (as well as Tillich) from a charge of outright unorthodoxy. Nonetheless, as Hume continues to remind us, the convenient binary opposition between "atheist" and "Christian" is far from stable, and my examples from the ancient world, the Middle Ages, and our own times can show something of how persistently this is the case. In this context it might be worth remembering, if only in passing, that in traditions such as Buddhism and Taoism, the problem scarcely exists in the form of a binary opposition in the first place.

For historical reasons, then, the word "atheist" bears no single sense, but its value as a descriptive term can be questioned for other reasons as well. For instance, "atheist" has the word "god" already inscribed within it, so that an unbeliever is co-opted by the believer's discourse before discussion even begins. Not surprisingly, some participants in a survey designed to assess the end-of-life needs of atheists objected to the use of the term, and preferred "'skeptics,' 'freethinkers,' or 'secular humanists.'" As Marilyn Smith-Stoner (2007, 927), who conducted the survey, concludes (slightly sheepishly), "the term 'atheist' may need revising."

I will be brief in turning from atheism to agnosticism, which is also a prescribed part of my topic. As Michael Martin (2007, 1) points out, "an atheist is someone without belief in God; he or she need not be someone who believes that God does not exist." However, some atheists do believe that God does not exist, and the term is usually understood in this second, more combative, sense. Martin also notices that atheism understood in the first sense overlaps with agnosticism in so far as agnostics are without belief in God, basing their position on the claim that human knowledge is not fitted to determine whether God exists or not.

As is well known, the term "agnostic" in its modern sense is the invention of T. H. Huxley (1825–1895), though the Greek word *agnostos* is as old as Homer. Huxley became embroiled in much lively controversy with theologians, and, as a result, agnosticism was associated especially with his claim that there is insufficient evidence for God's existence. But for Huxley, agnosticism as a matter of principle reaches further, as he makes clear:

> This principle may be stated in various ways, but they all amount to this: that it is wrong for a man to say that he is certain of the objective truth of any proposition unless he can produce evidence which logically justifies that certainty. This is what Agnosticism asserts; and, in my opinion, it is all that is essential to Agnosticism. (Huxley 1889, 309)

This passage sets out a position that applies to knowledge in general, and not just to theology. And so, as with the word "atheist," we can distinguish between a narrow and a broad sense of "agnostic," and it is easy to see how the different senses of both terms can overlap, allowing for a wide range of nuances.

I have set out these concerns because I want to suggest that caregivers preparing to attend to dying atheists or agnostics should at the very least have thought such things through so that they will know why and how to tread carefully. All of which can bring us back to the two poems with which I began. In both, as we see, a personal voice speaks to us, engaging us beyond what "Christian" and "atheist" alone can tell us. In short, there is an elision between what the poems say and the descriptive labels that the authors would willingly apply to themselves. I want to propose that this elision is exactly the place where a conversation with another person (whether at the end of life or otherwise) becomes most authentic and efficacious.

I am not going to dwell on "spirituality," the third main concept that guides the discussion in each of our chapters. The growing prevalence of the term in the literature of end-of-life care is documented by other contributors, and the problems raised by a simplistic opposition between "spirituality" and "religion" is also sufficiently noticed elsewhere in this collection. Broadly, the assumption that by virtue of being human we are "spiritual," as stated, for instance by Bradshaw (1996, 415) and widely replicated throughout the field of end-of-life care, is frequently tendentious.

Certainly, in the literature with which I am familiar, sentences in which the word "spiritual" occurs are often stronger if the word is omitted. For instance, Randall and Downie (2006, 165) describe counseling as "spiritual care" if "the latter is taken as helping a person in search of meaning." Spiritual care, here, is counseling in disguise, and, besides, is nothing more than helping someone to find meaning. In her excellent contribution to the present collection, Kathleen Garces-Foley cites Shirley Smith's advice about how to get a "spiritual" conversation going by asking questions such as, "What is especially meaningful or frightening to you now?" This might indeed be a way to get a conversation going, but I have had at least one dying friend on whom I could count to reply: "The war in

Afghanistan." Neither the question nor this answer strikes me as "spiritual," unless, as with Randall and Downie, the word is trivialized to mean something like "meaningful exchange." In a telling moment of reflection, Marilyn Smith-Stoner (who, you will recall, had second thoughts about the word "atheist") ducks for cover again when some of her surveyed atheists objected also to the term "spiritual." "Use of the term 'spiritual,'" she suggests, "may be most appropriate for team members in discussing care, rather than with the patient and family, unless an effort is made to clarify the contextual meaning of the term" (2007, 927). The notion that end-of-life caregivers should use "spiritual" as a code word, concealed from patients and families, exhibits an embarrassment in print that the author is at pains otherwise to conceal.

Still, to be fair, the last part of Smith-Stoner's sentence—about finding an agreement on what the term means in a specific context—does make good sense, and despite the impatience I have displayed in the preceding remarks, I do not in principle object to each and every use of "spiritual" and its cognates. Nonetheless, it is better to avoid the kind of imprecision that empties the word of content by failing to discriminate among its different but allied senses, for instance in theology (spirit indicating the supernatural life of grace), philosophical theology (spirit opposed to matter), and philosophy (Hegel's subjective, objective, and absolute spirit). Once we know what language game is being played, it can make sense to conceive even of an "atheist spirituality," as carefully described, for instance, by André Comte-Sponville (2007, 134). All of which brings me to a key distinction toward which this discussion has steadily been moving.

As we see, terms such as "atheist," "agnostic," and "spiritual" do tell us something, and can be useful. But there is a difference between what is sometimes called a "real definition" and a "nominal definition." For instance, language cannot provide a real definition of God, except with such a high degree of abstraction as to be virtually empty of content. Consequently, any useful conversation about God must settle for a nominal definition, which is to say, it must start by asking: "Tell me what you mean by God, and I'll tell you if I believe or not." Throughout the previous discussion, I have pointed to the difficulties attending real definitions of our key terms, but this is not to say that nominal definitions are not helpful. And so at this point I have put myself on the spot, if only because, as the editors say, the present chapter is supposed to reflect my own "atheist/agnostic perspective." This mandate combined with the course of the preceding argument suggests that I should now say what particular kind (if any) of atheist or agnostic I take myself to be, and what difference this might make to what I think about end-of-life care.

And so, here it is. I do not believe that there is a creator God who, somehow, stands above and beyond the universe, bringing it into being by fiat and then watching over it, responsive to prayer, willing to intervene in miraculous ways, and declaring a special revelation that is enshrined in books, which are then held sacred. On the agnostic front, I agree with T. H. Huxley that there is insufficient evidence for the kind of God I have described here, but I also have a special fondness for the more general aspect of agnosticism that Huxley espouses. That is, I believe we are all agnostics when it comes to the question: What happens after we die? No one knows, and the world's major religions should begin by acknowledging that they don't know either. As a corollary, I believe that sacred books, like all books, are written by humans, and according them an extraordinary, sacrosanct status arises mainly from political considerations. This does not mean that I do not find such books interesting and often compelling, but for me they mainly share these qualities with other works of literature.

I find value also in a wide range of religious traditions and practices. For instance, in certain circumstances religion can offer a progressive critique of political power structures, and a well-regulated religious observance can be psychologically salutary. Here I part company with "new atheists" such as Christopher Hitchins and Richard Dawkins, and I prefer the political critique of the Marxist Terry Eagleton and the cultural critique informing the "atheist spirituality" of André Comte-Sponville. Still, in so far as the new atheists draw attention to the undeniably toxic aspects of religion, I applaud them for doing so.

Finally, I do not think that the positions I have set out are merely negative; rather, I experience them as liberating. As the atheist philosopher Derek Parfit explains:

When I changed my view, the walls of my glass tunnel disappeared. I now live in the open air. There is still a difference between my life and the lives of other people. But the difference is less. Other people are closer. I am less concerned about the rest of my own life, and more concerned about the lives of others. (1987, 281)

In his interesting article "Atheists: A Psychological Profile" (2007, 313), Benjamin Beit-Hallahmi concludes that, for reasons resembling those set out by Parfit, atheists, far from being negative and depressive, are, in fact, likely to be tolerant and conscientious and are "good to have as neighbors." Amen to that.

And so, my cards are on the table. But the problem is that my cards are not just those displayed in the immediately preceding paragraphs on what atheism and agnosticism mean to me. Rather, they are everything I have said so far, and here we return to the point I wanted to make by citing those two poems. "Atheist" and "Christian," "unbeliever" and "believer" do not tell us enough about the personal statements that encompass and transfigure the labels we apply—not incorrectly—to their authors. Just so, even my own account of how it is not incorrect to describe me as a certain variety of atheist and agnostic does not tell you as much about what and how I think as do the preceding pages taken together. The question is, how would you describe the differences between the paragraphs describing my nominal atheism and the text of this essay as a whole? That, again, is the elision that, I suggest, needs to be entered into to make further conversation meaningful rather than trivial, engaged rather than superficial. When a person is dying, a caregiver will, I presume, try for the meaningful and engaged. What does it take, then, to inhabit the elision, to humanize the dehumanizing pathos and wretchedness of the dying body?

"IT'S NOT ALL RIGHT": OURSELVES AT THE LIMIT

In the literature I have read on the topic, there is general agreement that good palliative care is the place to begin. The provision of physical comfort to the extent that this is attainable opens a space for whatever further interventions might ease the fears, anxieties, and other concerns that can trouble a dying person. An account of the knowledge and skill requisite for good medical practice is beyond the scope of what I have to say here. But, for instance, such an account is provided in impressive detail by Joseph Fins (2006), who brings to bear his medical expertise in assessing the complexities of palliative medication, including such topics as legal constraints, futility disputes, surrogate decision making, withdrawal of care, and the right to die. Making a patient as comfortable as can be managed by medical intervention, even when no cure is in the offing, is clearly a priority, and it is consoling to know that the range of expertise described by Fins is available at least to some of those in need of it. The task then is for caregivers to assess what kinds of further attention might help to minimize the anguish and emotional pain of dying—including the complex ways in which emotional pain can manifest as physical pain.

As an aid to such assessment, "spiritual needs charts" and "assessment tools" are sometimes deployed. Commentators tend to mention these to dismiss them as "cumbersome" or "burdensome" (Kuebler et al. 2005, 326) or even as expressing a "paternalism" based on "delusion" (Randall and Downie 2006, 20). Still, I can imagine that, in the right hands, a careful list of questions might help to indicate the kind of assistance that would be of most benefit to a dying patient. Nonetheless, reading a "spiritual needs chart" and reading, say, a poem are so utterly different as to be all but mutually exclusive, and given that I am using poetry to highlight the irreducible significance of the personal voice, I would want to see even the best spiritual needs chart go into the bottom drawer before any real, engaged conversation begins. Certainly, a chart that might designate a person "atheist" or "agnostic" would tell us too little, and, as I have suggested, a caregiver needs to know in advance about the range of complexities that attend such descriptive labels. For instance, there can be greater incompatibility among different kinds of atheists than among some atheists and some believers. Repeatedly, I find myself stumbling upon the awkward truth that I have more in common with many thoughtful believers than those same believers have with their own more literal-minded coreligionists.

After all, the next atheist you meet might be a version of Shakespeare's Barnardine in *Measure for Measure*, who, sentenced to death and about to be executed, simply doesn't care and exhibits a splendid, unrepentant, drunken defiance. Barnardine is impervious to every appeal that he should pray and repent. He is "careless, reckless, and fearless of what's past, present, or to come" (IV, 2, 146–47), as the appalled Provost tells the Duke, and indeed there is something horrifying in his sheer, insensate ferocity. Yet Barnardine is a welcome relief from the religious neurotics surrounding him. They are much more toxic than he is, their humanity distorted by their religious principles gone wrong. As ever, Shakespeare calculates the effect unerringly.

But the next atheist you meet might not be like Barnardine at all, but rather a version, say, of Dostoevsky's Ivan Karamazov, who declares his unbelief to his brother, the young monk Alyosha, by way of the legend of the Grand Inquisitor in *The Brothers Karamazov*. This conversation between the brothers is one of the subtlest yet also most confrontational explorations of unbelief in print anywhere. As a careful reader discovers, the interplay between the dramatic context of Ivan's conversation and his deliberately provocative poem about the Grand Inquisitor is highly intricate, and Ivan's position—on the surface so blasphemous and contemptuous of the God who would allow the suffering of children—is in fact shot through with difficulties and obscurities in which readers soon find themselves disturbingly entangled.

One reason Ivan is complicated is because his is what we might call a protest atheism. That is, he is reacting against the religion that has shaped his thinking and sensibility, and, not surprisingly, the results are fraught and equivocal. By contrast, Barnardine's atheism is an atheism of indifference. He doesn't want to discuss the topic because he has no interest in it. Among the atheists and agnostics I have met, many more are like Ivan than like Barnardine, for whom spiritual care makes sense only if it comes out of a bottle. We might recall that the word "spirits," as applied to liquor, derives from Galenic medicine, where spirits are thin vapors mediating between body and soul. For what it is worth, I would feel inclined to give Barnardine his medicine, which is to say, the spiritual care he says he wants.

Ivan is much more problematic, if only because protest atheism is not straightforward. Also, unlike the dumbfounding Barnardine, Ivan is too clever for his own good, and might well enjoy, for instance, giving a caregiver a difficult time. There is no telling what unlikely turns a discussion with the Ivans of this world might take, and it is not surprising to learn that a significant number of self-described secularists reengage their early religious convictions when they are near death (Hart 1994). Whether they do so because they are conflicted, as Ivan is, or are rediscovering a dimension of the old religion that they value after all, or because their faculties are failing and they are no longer lucid might not be easy to say. Nonetheless, an effective caregiver needs to be able not only to separate the Barnardines from the Ivans, but also to assess the numerous ways in which the attitudes represented by Barnardine and Ivan might overlap and mingle.

Here again we return to the irreducible complexity of persons, and, for reasons that I have set out, I am not comfortable describing this complexity simply as "spiritual." The phrase "whole person care," which is also current in the literature, strikes me as a better choice, and I expect that those nonbelievers who objected to the words "atheist" and "spiritual" would be less bothered by care being directed to them as "whole persons."

Michael Kearney's long experience as a doctor in the hospice movement leads him to recommend a combination of palliative medicine and educated discernment of the specific needs of individual persons. Thus, he proposes that "the combined approach of multi professional expertise and compassionate attention to the whole person" is an ideal worth aspiring to, especially given the fact that "total pain" prevents clear distinctions among the different kinds of intervention that caregivers can provide (1997, 17). Yet Kearney's focus on whole person care has a corollary that can easily be neglected but in my view is of pressing significance.

That is, Kearney insists on the limitations of what caregivers can do. We need to accept that we cannot make things right, that death is the ultimate separation, and the fact that "it's hard and horrible" (106) means that we are human. We don't have the answer for a distraught sufferer who insists, "It's not all right" (126), and we need to understand that healer and patient share a common wound—namely, their mortality. When it comes to the final reckoning, we are "human . . . with human" (56), and not only should a dying patient try to let go the ego structures by which control is exerted, but so should the healer. The uncomfortable fact is that a doctor's helplessness in face of the incurable wound can stimulate a fight or flight reaction, resulting either in the ill-advised imposition of further treatments or a panic-stricken retreat from the scene, disguised, for instance, as handing the patient over to a different kind of caregiver (65–66). Kimberley Patton (2009, 7) makes the point more bluntly, claiming that many doctors actually dislike seriously ill people: "The truth is that they want to get away from them." She cites Jerome Groopman's *How Doctors Think* (2007) to comment further on the consequences of this unfortunate aversion.

I have no idea about the extent to which Patton's claim is true, but she does echo in a suggestive way the points raised by Kearney about fear in the face of helplessness. All of which in turn has a bearing on a central assertion in the main line of atheist literature from, let us say, Lucretius to Freud, declaring that we should accept the fact that life is irreducibly tragic. As Kearney says, our mortal wound is beyond healing and we need to acknowledge this difficult truth (together with its corollary, I would want to say, that we don't know what happens after we die). Accepting the tragic realities of death, ignorance, and our final helplessness—without attempting to sugar the pill—might help, in turn, to take us beyond the defenses erected by the ego to evade these hard facts. Yet neither do I think that a tragic sense of life precludes joy, delight, wonder, compassion, and the kind of liberation described by Parfit, whereby "other people are closer" and we are more concerned about their lives and less about our own. Rather, a tragic sense of life is likely to call forth defiance or protest (such as we see in Ivan), and a well-tempered combination of defiance and compassion is, to me, an expression of human solidarity that I would hope to find in a caregiver, not just at life's end, but at any time at all.

If it seems contradictory to recommend defiance on the one hand and egoless acceptance on the other, I would suggest that accepting something and condoning it are not the same. Again, literature can show especially well how a balance between these apparently contrary impulses might be effected as a lived experience. Anyone who is curious might profitably spend time in the company of Dr. Rieux in Albert Camus' remarkable novel, *The Plague*. For now, I want only to notice that the clarity with which the likes of Lucretius, Spinoza, Nietzsche, and Camus face life's tragedy, unconsoled by the benign providential solicitude of a creator God while at the same time declaring a defiantly radical affirmation—"the eternal Yea," as Carlyle says—is a testament to what is best in us, standing alongside, together.

CONCLUSION: OF PERSONS AND CULTURES

I am now pretty much at the end of what I have to say, but I have not yet considered how an adequate education could be provided for end-of-life caregivers to learn what I am suggesting they need to know to be of best assistance to people who might share the kinds of views and commitments I have been setting out here. The "multi professional" ideal described by Kearney has been quite widely implemented, and it is not unusual for counselors, massage therapists, artists in residence, dream analysts, chaplains, guided imagery practitioners, and so on to be available to patients in hospice care. Still, there is a difference between co-opting nonmedical kinds of knowledge and modifying the education of the medical practitioners themselves. In the United Kingdom, Special Study Modules are now available within the medical curriculum to allow students to develop particular interests and capacities through approved studies in humanities subjects as well as other areas of science. As Randall and Downie (2006, 200) point out, "palliative medicine claims to alleviate emotional, psychological, social, and spiritual suffering, in addition to physical symptoms. There is no other specialty which claims to do all these." Without compromising the integrity of the core curriculum, an appropriate cultivation of special aptitudes and talents might well awaken new kinds of humane understanding that can have highly practical applications within this especially complex field. After all, a single drop of dye can change the complexion of an entire vial of clear liquid.

In this context, it is worth remembering that attention to the "whole person" entails—however tacitly—the presence of a "whole culture," if only because person and culture are mutually interdependent and mirror each another. As Northrop Frye (1963, 66) points out, education "affects the whole person, not bits and pieces of him. It doesn't just train the mind; it's a social and moral development too." In the same study, Frye points out that highly developed science and art are closely allied (6–7), and this being the case, as I believe it is, the best of science-based medicine and the best compassionate attention and understanding should converge as the expression of a humane culture at large, within which the best insights and practices are developed as a matter of general education and not only as a specialty confined to the terminally ill. This of course is a utopian view, but like other ideals of the kind, it can help to direct our aspirations as long as we do not require of human beings that they attain a perfection of which they are incapable.

As I hope to have shown, atheism and agnosticism are inscribed within such a total view in complex ways, carrying their own challenges and exerting their own critical force in relation to more mainline religious beliefs and practices. Those who might find themselves caring for a dying atheist need, in advance, to know how to read such complexities—as with the voices of the two poems with which I began. With this in mind, I am drawn, in conclusion, to a point made by the cultural theorist Slavoj Žižek (1997, 50), who reminds us that none of us is ever quite as we are defined, and we remain to some degree opaque to ourselves and to one another. Something escapes, and that absence—what I have referred to as an elision—is, paradoxically, our best opportunity for meeting one another authentically. That is, the inarticulate in itself summons a recognition at once tragic and compassionate, beyond the consolations that can be given a voice. Yet neither does such recognition dispense with the voice that, taken to its limit, acknowledges the deeper human claim that always escapes it, and which, once recognized, can then also inform what might be spoken.

As I said at the start, I offer these remarks as an outsider to the expertise that makes a highly admirable, immediate difference to people's lives every day through the provision of end-of-life care. But in so far as such expertise is also the expression of larger cultural values without which the expertise itself cannot very well survive or even come into being, an outsider's voice putting the case for a minority view might perhaps strike a harmonious note after all, resonant in proportion to its unexpectedness.

Still, as a last word, I remain curious. Which poem did you say was written by the Christian, and which by the atheist? And (more important) what were your reasons?

NOTES

1. The first poem is Christina Rosetti's (1830–1894) "Uphill." The second is from A. E. Housman's (1859–1936) A Shropshire Lad, in which many poems are untitled. This is number L, which, instead of a title, has the following header:

Clunton and Clunbury,
   Clungford and Clun,
Are the quietest places
   Under the sun

REFERENCES

Beit-Hallahmi, B. 2007. Atheists: A psychological profile. The Cambridge companion to atheism. Cambridge: Cambridge University Press.

Bradshaw, A. 1996. The spiritual dimension of hospice: The secularization of an ideal. Social Science & Medicine 43(3): 401–19.

Comte-Sponville, A. 2007. The little book of atheist spirituality. New York: Viking.

Dostoevsky, F. 1982. The brothers Karamazov. London: Penguin.

Fins, J. J. 2006. A palliative ethic of care: Clinical wisdom at life's end. Boston: James and Bartlett.

Frye, N. 1963. *The educated imagination*. Toronto: Canadian Broadcasting Corporation.

Groopman, J. 2007. *How doctors think*. Boston: Houghton Mifflin.

Hart, C. W. 1994. Spiritual health, illness, and death. *Journal of Religion and Health* 33(1): 17–22.

Hume, D. 1779. *Dialogues concerning natural religion*. London.

Huxley, T. H. 1889. *Agnosticism and Christianity: Science and Christian tradition*. New York: D. Appleton.

Justin Martyr. 1884 (reprinted 1996). *The first apology*. Edinburgh: T. and T. Clark, 159ff.

Kearney, M. 1997. *Mortally wounded*. New York: Simon and Schuster.

Kuebler, K., K. Davis, P. Mellar, and C. D. Moore. 2005. *Palliative practices: An interdisciplinary approach*. Maryland Heights, MO: Elsevier Mosby.

Martin, M. 2007. General introduction. *The Cambridge companion to atheism*. Cambridge: Cambridge University Press.

Meister Eckhart. 1924. *Meister Eckhart*. London: John Watkins.

Parfit, D. 1987. *Reasons and persons*. Oxford: Clarendon Press.

Patton, K. C. 2009. Ancient Asklepieia: Institutional incubation and the hope of healing. In *Imagination and medicine: The future of healing in an age of neuroscience*, ed. S. Aizenstat and R. Bosnak. New Orleans: Spring Journal, 3–34.

Randall, F., and R. S. Downie. 2006. *The philosophy of palliative care: Critique and reconstruction*. Oxford: Oxford University Press.

Shakespeare, W.. 1972. *Measure for measure. The complete Signet Shakespeare*. New York: Harcourt Brace.

Smith-Stoner, M. 2007. End-of-life preferences for atheists. *Journal of Palliative Medicine* 10(4): 923–28.

Ryland, J. E., trans. 1994. Introductory note to *Tatian the Assyrian*. In *Ante-Nicene Fathers*, volume 2, ed. A. Roberts and J. Donaldson. Peabody, MA: Hendrickson Publishers.

Tillich, P. 1973. *Systematic theology*. Chicago: Chicago University Press.

Žižek, S. 1997. *The abyss of freedom/ages of the world*. Ann Arbor: University of Michigan Press.

CHAPTER 7

Spirituality Unhinged

ELIZABETH CAUSTON

JUST AS PATRICK GRANT began his personal reflection with poetry, I am drawn to do the same, because I find that poetry, like life, can be rich with subtle nuances and ambiguities that encourage subjective interpretation, the search for constantly evolving meaning, and the opportunity for being surprised over and over again by new ways of seeing something familiar.

In his book *Mortally Wounded*, Michael Kearney (1996, 151) says that "the dying process midwifes a person into depth," invoking for me the image of a natural but mysterious journey in which we are pulled by internal gravity from the outer world down to that "incorruptible spot of grace at our core" so beautifully described by Mark Nepo (2006). These are a journey and a place best described by the language of symbolism and imagery.

So a poem that I have come to love, which will be read at my funeral just after the bagpipes play, is Mary Oliver's "In Blackwater Woods" (2003, 72–73). At the end of the poem, the author describes the glorious yet supremely paradoxical nature of being human when she says,

To live in this world

you must be able
to do three things:

to love what is mortal;
to hold it

against your bones knowing
Your own life depends on it;
and, when the time comes to let it go,
to let it go.

In my interpretation of this poem, we are called upon to acknowledge that there are many things we will never know, and in recognizing this, discover we can get on with doing the "three things" needed for living well in this world. This concept is important to me, because instead of trying to define where I am on the spiritual-religious continuum, it allows me to express that which I would most want you to know about me when I am dying: that I have loved "what is mortal"; that I have "held it against my bones," knowing with absolute certainty that everything that life means to me depends on it; and that I fear letting those beloved mortals go more than anything on earth—that getting through that goodbye will be the hardest thing I ever do.

I also want you to know that I wouldn't have it any other way. I believe the pain of separation in death validates the courage it takes to love in this way. So my hope is that no one will try to comfort me with platitudes about seeing my loved ones again in a heavenly afterlife, or attempt to minimize either my "emotional" or my "spiritual pain" by helping me to "resolve" my grief. When I die, I will not hold those I love against my bones again. For me this will be an "unfixable" pain, unresponsive to the attempts at amelioration that so often appear to be the goal of both medicine and religion in the care of the dying.

This is not to say that I don't believe that good pain control should not be offered for intractable symptoms at end of life. However, having worked in a hospice setting for fourteen years, I saw many situations in which physical suffering could not be fully relieved even with the most skillful palliative care, and even more instances where emotional pain and grief proved to be untreatable. I also observed that in the presence of such intractable pain, the inclination was for health care professionals to *do* more: more assessments and evaluations to try and figure out the etiology of the pain, followed by more experiments with different medications and therapies to try and "fix" it. Because of this tendency, I worry that by dying in the context of the Western hero/victim medical model described so clearly by Michael Kearney (1996), I could become the "victim" of "heroes" whose need to rescue me both physically and spiritually will overshadow my own needs and wishes, especially if they are, as I suspect they will be, complicated, difficult to articulate, and even contradictory at times.

Of course, the problem with this pervasive emphasis on "doing" is that attention often shifts away from the patient to trying to determine who among all the different "specialists" has the best skills to "get the job done." This creates an atmosphere of competition between health care disciplines that is ultimately destructive and self-serving. I am troubled by the lack of interdisciplinary respect and generosity that too often characterizes not only the delivery of palliative care, but of health care in general. I believe that there is far too much internal arguing about "ownership" of areas of perceived expertise, with the result that chaplains claim to be the best—if not the ones solely qualified—to talk about religious issues, nurses claim to epitomize the embodiment of the holistic approach, and social workers and counselors jealously guard psychosocial care.

These developments are disturbing at two levels. First, the superficial division of labor reflected in the need to know definitively whether the dying patient is experiencing "emotional," "spiritual," or "psychosocial" distress creates a false and, for the patient, often confusing sense of division between these different domains. Second, it appears that the very clinicians whose mandate in health care is to work with, but not within, our problem-focused medical model have embraced this labeling process precisely in order to analyze and then *do* something about people's spiritual "problems." Surely we must be willing to ask how these labels, which reduce human experiences, values, and beliefs to one- or two-word sound bites, actually help to provide better care at end of life. And how is the need to know whether distress is emotional or spiritual different from the tendency among medical specialists to effectively divide the human body into its smallest parts so that the "right" specialist can lay claim to the physical territory that "belongs" to them? I would argue that this tendency toward division and labeling, though convenient in the moment, fails to acknowledge and therefore validate the inherently holistic nature of human beings and their lived experience.

In this light, it is perhaps instructive to point to how the research documented in the other chapters of this book suggests that the first choice of many dying people as to whom they feel most comfortable talking with about their spiritual issues is family and friends. So while clinicians hover and jockey for the right to intervene, one might imagine the patient having a deep and meaningful conversation with a loved one who is not concerned with the question of whether their distress is emotional or spiritual. Might this not imply that the quality of the relationship is more important than a particular professional title; or that shared personal history is more important than expertise; or that having a meaningful conversation is more important than getting answers or being "fixed"? Nonmedical clinicians ought to consider balancing the specialization and scientific approach that characterizes the medical model with a holistic approach that focuses less on separation and more on seeking out the stories and personal historical contexts that will help them better understand the meaning of pain, death, and separation for a particular individual at a given time. In order to do this, however, clinicians must approach patients and families as explorers, not just as detectives.

When health care professionals listen as detectives, they listen for facts such as the location, severity, and quality of someone's physical pain. Detectives always have a puzzle they are trying to solve with the result that new information is categorized as useful or irrelevant depending upon how it fits into a preconceived pattern. Medical detectives often cut people off when they wander from the facts; their work is driven by questions they feel obligated to ask, and they become frustrated with people who struggle to articulate, let alone change, their answers. The point of the detective's job is to eliminate the unknown, and they are unlikely to be satisfied until that is accomplished.

However, listening as an explorer involves a willingness to go into uncharted territory and to be surprised by what might be around the next bend; it means approaching the journey without preconceived ideas based on predetermined labels or diagnoses. It means being open-minded and willing to be and even remain "unknowing," asking open-ended questions that allow patients and families to share what they believe, value, and cherish as well as what they fear and hope for. And then it means resisting the need to classify people's answers and recognizing that, just like an ever-changing landscape, human beings are never static but in constant motion at every level of their being. Whereas the unknown is a challenge or even a source of discomfort for the detective, it is the explorer's source of joy, well within their comfort zone.

Much of medicine is like detective work, and while there is no question this is often both appropriate and necessary, nonmedical clinicians must constantly be mindful of the temptation to get caught up in a similar "need to know" mentality that may lead to forgetting how to just "be" in the presence of the unknown as it is epitomized by death.

So, when I am dying and struggling with that last goodbye, I want to be approached by an explorer, a fellow traveler facing the same unknown as I am; someone who is able to be surprised and delighted by ideas, beliefs, and mysteries that she or he could never have imagined. I want to be visited by someone like Wayne Muller, who, although an ordained minister, approaches the dying person as nothing more (or less) than "one who will also die" (1996, 274). From a place of deep humility and caring, and without any personal or professional agenda, Wayne Muller waits for and trusts the process as it unfolds:

> When I sit with the dying, I do not really do anything at all. I sit without expectation. I listen, I hold their hand, I let them cry. I really cannot do anything "significant." I cannot cure their disease. I cannot save their life. I cannot take away their pain. I cannot make them not be alone at night. I cannot "do" anything.
>
> So why do they ask for me? I believe that it is because for a few moments, in the quiet of our shared company they can finally hear themselves. . . . They

speak to me of what they love, and they remember what
is important. This moment is not about medicines, and
treatments and diagnoses and prognoses. It is about
how it feels to be alive and yet only for this short time.
And I, one who will also die, sit and wait with them.
We wait together. (1996, 274)

Likewise, in her beautiful book of stories, *Kitchen Table
Wisdom*, Rachel Remen (1997) offers us exquisite examples of
listening and of her willingness to be led by those she "companions" and guides in the dying process. Distinguishing
between the concepts of healing and curing, she defines healing
as something that happens when a person feels that they have
been "seen and heard and validated" (Rachel Remen, personal
communication), meaning that healing can happen even when
a cure is no longer possible. When I am dying, I will want a
listener and a healer at my bedside, not a fixer or a fighter, and
certainly not someone telling me not to be afraid because the
next life will be better. What Remen and Muller have in common, what all healers have in common, is an ability to be fully
present to the human being before them, in the moment, with
an open heart and a generosity of spirit that allows them to
listen as a compassionate witness, knowing that that may be
exactly what is needed. It may be, in fact all that is needed.

Listening is the oldest and perhaps the most powerful
tool of healing. When we listen, we offer with our attention, an opportunity for wholeness. Our listening creates sanctuary for the homeless parts within the other
person: that which has been denied, unloved, devalued
by themselves and by others; that which may have been
hidden. Listening creates a holy silence. When you listen
generously to people, they can hear the truth in themselves, often for the first time. (Remen 1996, 219–20)

The question I ask in the context of this chapter is, am I
unique in this wish to be listened to and, by Rachel Remen's
definition, to be healed? Or is this a universal human need that
has become overlooked in the push to emphasize how people

are different from each other? I was asked to write this reflection from the perspective of someone who is "spiritual but not religious," as if that category defines a homogeneous yet separate group of people whose needs at the end of life will somehow be different from those who define themselves as religious or, at the other end of the continuum, not spiritual at all. I still wonder, however, even as I fill the pages with my ideas and concerns, if this distinction will serve me well when I am dying. At the end of the day (or life) will it matter what "box" or category I fit into, or, since all boxes are equally constraining, will any box only serve to separate me from my fellow human beings as well as from the complexity of who I really am?

So, when I half-jokingly described myself to the other authors as "spiritual but not religious except when I'm not spiritual," I was really saying that I don't want to be put into a box, especially if that box gives someone just enough information to think they can make the sweeping assumptions that labels invite them to make about who I am, what I believe (or don't believe!), and what is or is not missing in my life. The fact is that I have many "homeless parts" that remain difficult to articulate, much less categorize. However, rather than creating a sanctuary, a safe place for these "homeless parts" to rest, I sense a need in our care of the dying to resolve and repair this "homeless" state. When this has been achieved, one can almost hear the collective sigh of relief that a suitable "home" has been located, the conflicting and confusing beliefs cleared out, and the dying person moved to a comfortable and coherent space . . . one more person saved in the nick of time from the streets of ambivalence and spiritual homelessness.

In his thought-provoking article "Searching Self-Image: Identities to Be Self-Evident," James Haywood Rolling (2004) speaks eloquently about the sense of homelessness a person might experience when they cannot classify themselves or be classified by others into a neatly defined and widely accepted category:

> Homelessness is a terrible thing to have to admit. It renders unclassifiable those who occupy its murky stations. Without an acceptable address, how can I prove

my legitimacy? And yet the state of homelessness is an important launching point for the following [question]: . . . Can I be myself if I cannot see my sheltering framework, if I do not know where I live, if I cannot entirely discern or speak my ideological address? (2004, 870)

In my own spiritual journey of consciously choosing to become spiritually homeless, at least for the time being, I not only believe that I am indeed "being myself," but that like Rolling, "in spite of the inadequacy of classifications, I am clearly more than has been previously stated" (2004, 871). However, having said that, there was a time when I did inhabit a well-known spiritual structure, and leaving that home has involved a long, often lonely, and not always easy or comfortable quest to rediscover and rename myself. Rolling reflects on the ultimate value of this endeavor:

Naming can alternatively be a definition of identity or a source of stigma. Un-naming can alter a story and serve to unhinge fixed definitions, initiating a democratic discourse that finds its own way of escaping the thrall of hegemony and dominating canons. (2004, 869)

Rachel Remen (1997) also writes about the impact of the judgments that so often accompany this process of naming and identifying: "The life in us is diminished by judgment far more frequently than by disease. Our own self-judgment or the judgment of other people can stifle our life force, its spontaneity and natural expression" (35). "Life is as complex as we are," she says. "It is not an either/or world. It is a real world. In calling ourselves 'heads' or 'tails,' we may never own and spend our human currency, the pure gold of which our coin is made" (38).

As I have become more unhinged from fixed definitions, I have also become more whole and, in the process, discovered a spiritual "home away from home" with movable walls and no fixed address. However, this has not always been the case. My original spiritual identity was as a Lutheran, and a specific kind of Lutheran at that. As a young adult, filled with doubt and skepticism, I rebelled against the restrictions of my upbringing by becoming an Anglican, which of course was more of a lateral move than a huge religious or philosophical shift. It was finally in my mid-forties that I read and found a temporary sanctuary in the writings of Sam Keen, discovering through him that "the doubt I despised was a treasure that would enrich me in the absence of faith" (1994, 79). The idea that doubt could be a treasure opened a forbidden door in my spiritual home, and I never looked back.

Next came Harold Kushner (1983) and his book *When Bad Things Happen to Good People*, with his stunning revelation that one could not see the world clearly and still believe that God could be compassionate and just as well as all-powerful. Something had to give, and for Kushner, it was his belief in an all-powerful God. Nothing that I had ever read in the Bible, been taught as a child, or experienced in my life to that time made more sense than his reworking of a deeply troubling equation that had challenged my common sense while creating a crisis of faith that I had tried for so long to ignore. What I valued most about Kushner, however, was that when he wrote his book his only concern was making sense of his son's death in his own personal world. If his perspective helped others come to grips with tragedies that made no sense in their own lives then that was fine with him. But his greatest need was to find a way to survive the loss of his son while maintaining a belief in a God he could still turn to for divine strength and compassion. In other words, he kept what was important to him in his understanding of the world, remaining true to his deepest convictions, while letting go of a belief that no longer supported his personal experience of life. While this revised belief system, which felt holistic and coherent to Kushner, did not need to make sense to anyone else, the fact that it actually resonated with hundreds of thousands of people who read his book did not ultimately determine his belief in the rightness of this "new theology" for himself.

Kushner's search for personal meaning is not fundamentally different from what has motivated and continues to motivate me to engage in a dynamic and evolving process of spiritual seeking, finding, and seeking yet again, although my quest will likely involve a different ending than his. Of course there are people who have known the home that is right for them from birth, and those who have sought out and found their spiritual home in a community of like-minded believers. Obviously, homelessness or the spiritually nomadic lifestyle is not for everyone, and not everyone who is homeless in this way is on the same journey or looking for the same place to settle down.

Many years ago I encountered through my hospice work an elderly woman who had been living on the street for most of her adult life. I remember approaching her with profound assumptions about what it meant to be "homeless." Smugly, I "empathized" with her misfortune of having no worldly possessions and of not belonging to a community she could identify with. I judged her for lacking stability, for not taking responsibility, and for having to be dependent on others who had chosen a "better" lifestyle to keep "things going." I imagined her regret at not having had as full and rich a life as she could have had and her grief at having nothing to leave as a legacy. Fortunately she saved me from my smugness. She spoke of her freedom to be present to life and to the experiences and people she met without the distraction of things. She traveled light and could fit everything that was important to her in one small bag, the same small bag she brought to hospice, the sum total of all of her belongings. Her legacy was not in things but in memories, the ones she left with others as she generously gave gifts of her time and attention to those she cared for and loved. She didn't judge others for their choices and chose not to be defined by those who felt the need to judge her. She was serene in her dying, as I imagine she had been in much of her living, and this woman who many thought had nothing to offer gave me, freely and with no strings attached, a life lesson I have never forgotten.

At the same time, I knew I could not live her lifestyle, even after I learned to understand it better through her eyes. I need and cherish my physical home, and I thrive on the deep family connections that keep me in a state of eternal belonging. But spiritually I crave the ability to travel freely. I only want to be constrained by how much time I have to think, explore, read, search, ponder, and consider. My spiritual legacy will likely not involve too many answers, but I hope to leave those I love with some really good questions. "My spirit," as Sam Keen says, "like love, cannot be contained within the horizons of my mind. It soars above reason and swoops down into the chaos beneath rationality. It travels with its own passport and freely crosses the frontiers of the known and explainable world" (1994, 72).

When I encountered the homeless woman described here, that label inevitably came with assumptions attached to it because labels are always a place where curiosity stops and assumptions take over. Likewise, I think it's safe for me to imagine that the label "spiritual but not religious" conjures up certain assumptions about my own belief systems and world-view. One might, for example, assume that my worldview is framed by question marks . . . and they would, in fact, be right.

While I believe that there probably is something after this life, that belief is largely based on my acceptance of the sci-entific theory that energy never dissipates. However, the exact nature of this afterlife is an unknown to me; it remains one of those framing question marks, and for the time being, I am okay with that. What I do know is that the only afterlife I am willing to consider does not include something called heaven or hell or some kind of judgment or further categorizing of people as "saved" or "unsaved." In fact, I find the idea that the specter of a life after death might somehow influence my behavior in this life absurd.

As I stand on that threshold, it is entirely possible that I will be afraid of that unknown. I may fear the finality of death and the physical separation from loved ones. But answers, where I believe that answers don't exist, will not ease those fears. I may want and need a companion as I walk through the valley of the shadow of death, someone who with a similar awe and respect for the unknown will accompany me to the threshold, but no experts need apply.

The metaphor that perhaps best describes my philosophy about life after death is that of the explorer, who though she may wish for a guidebook as she approaches a new land, will not be stopped by the lack of one from going ashore, albeit with a combination of fear and excitement. She also knows that wishing for a guidebook and believing that one exists based on the musings of others who also have never gone are two very different things.

Another common assumption about someone who is not religious and only sometimes spiritual is that they don't pray. But I do pray; I can't help myself. And so it was with great delight that I read that Sam Keen (1994) also prays, although he doesn't believe in it. He just does it. In the religious household I grew up in, prayers at home were used to start our meals and end the day, and as with the church liturgy, there was a certain amount of comfort in the familiar routine based on the belief that some well-intentioned father figure was in charge of the world and listening with an ear to granting my wishes.

However, while I still find myself praying for the safety of those I love (and occasionally for a parking spot), I now recognize it as a wish as opposed to a belief that an all-powerful god might choose to save one of my daughters while taking the life of another mother's cherished child. Most of my prayers are actually "thank-yous," spoken out into the universe for favors received or wishes fulfilled. So, while Harold Kushner still prays for strength in a crisis to his not-all-powerful God, as I am dying I imagine that, as I have in the past, I will turn to my inner strength, plumbing the universal depths and to find the as-yet untapped resources available there. In this process, I am confident that I will not travel alone, because while I have strong opinions and a certain amount of clarity about the spiritual self I have struggled so hard to know and love, I have no need in life or in death to be a "lone ranger." Throughout my life, I have cherished the caring and support of family and good friends, and that won't change as I am dying. However, on that last journey, it will be the compassionate witness, the fellow traveler, and the healer among the professionals, friends, and family that I will turn to for love and support.

This brings me to a third assumption I find is often made about those who do not belong to a particular religious or spiritual community, and that is that they will lack a reliable community of support as they are dying. In fact, this is the source of one of my father's favorite lectures on what I have lost in drifting away from the church. Certainly the community of his faith has been there for him in the loss of my mother, sister, and brother-in-law and will be there for him as he faces his own death, lessening the burden on family members who live far away. But it is also a narrow definition of community that links its value so exclusively to a shared religious affiliation. Having said that, I am mindful in my spiritual journey of the loss of this one kind of community and the need to seek out and define "other" communities of friends to participate with me in a mutual commitment to "be there" for one another other as we face the crises of illness and death, along with the joys of aging, parenthood, and friendship. I am fortunate to belong to such a community of women who, while diverse in our spiritual beliefs, are united in our respect and caring for each other; the significance of this community in my life should not be underestimated.

The question I would pose to those who work with the dying is: How would you get to know these things about me? Certainly not through a survey or questionnaire or by asking me questions weighed down with implicit assumptions (what I call detective questions in disguise). These would be questions like: What are you afraid of? Have you thought about the meaning of your life? What remains unresolved for you? I would be much more likely to positively respond to questions such as: What's happening for you right now? What do you think would be helpful for us to know about you or what helps you to feel safe? What's important to you right now? These are questions that derive from a place of trust, respect, and valuing of who I am, of how I know myself, and of my capacity to know what is sacred and true for me, without assuming that any other person who describes themselves as spiritual but not religious will see or experience the world as I do.

Wayne Muller offers wise guidance for all clinicians:

> The best of therapy, like the best of spiritual practice, recognizes what is whole, strong, and wise within each of us. It is just like good medicine, which essentially relies on the body's own resources, using treatments that gently remind the body that it is capable of healing

itself. So too, do good emotional and spiritual practices [and I would say, therapies] allow us to remember who we are in our strongest, deepest sense. (1996, 60)

Finally, I want to return to the question of why spirituality and especially spiritual homelessness become such crucial issues at the time of death. As I thought about the title of the book and the association between dying and the importance of spirituality at the end of life, I found myself wondering why we care so much about an individual's spirituality at this particular time in health care when, in my experience, we don't seem to care about it at any other time. For example, over the last thirty years, although I have been in hospital for a miscarriage, the birth of two babies, and thyroid surgery, I was never once asked about my spirituality, my values, my thoughts on the meaning of life, any unresolved issues I might have had, or my views on an afterlife. And yet, in the practice of palliative care, which is defined in its most limited form as comfort care of the dying, issues of spirituality often take center stage. I'm not saying this is wrong, but it is interesting to ask why this is the case. If spirituality is inherent in all human beings, and if it is related to a search for meaning that is meant to be a lifelong journey, why is it only important to health care professionals at the very end of life and even then primarily in palliative care settings?

There are perhaps a couple of reasons for this. First, for the sake of argument, I would suggest it might be a side effect of palliative care being "born" in the context of a deeply religious environment. Given Cicely Saunders's strong religious convictions, there was quite naturally a perceived need for the dying to engage in a process of resolution, of coming to terms with death, and of making peace with their God while looking ahead to an afterlife that would be a better place. Even though Cicely Saunders was known for her religious tolerance, it's probably fair to assume that everyone in her hospice was expected to reflect on their spirituality and that spiritual homelessness was seen, at the very least, as an unfortunate state of affairs.

In addition, given the current feeling among spiritual care professionals that they are being gradually (or perhaps not so gradually) phased out of palliative care programs, or are often only peripherally involved, it is reasonable for those of us involved in palliative care, and who may one day be the recipients of palliative care, to reevaluate the role of spirituality in our approach to care of the dying. This is because our answers will determine not only *how* we ask people about spirituality at the end of life but, more importantly, *why* we ask them about spirituality as a separate category. What is our agenda, what resources do we assign to this aspect of care, and who (which profession) is considered to be the most qualified to deal with these issues?

I recall in my early days as a social worker struggling to find a way to acknowledge Kübler-Ross's groundbreaking work in putting "death on the table" while also accepting that her stages of grief did not accurately describe what we currently see as a much more nuanced and fluid process. Similarly, I believe that we can give Cicely Saunders credit for starting a revolution in care of the dying while letting go of her deeply religious model of care without being afraid that in doing so we will have lost the essence of good palliative care.

While there is a place for hospices funded by religious institutions that accept and serve individuals who ascribe to a particular faith, I am not in favor of returning to a religious model of hospice care. Nor do I believe that spiritual/religious resources should be funded more aggressively than social work and other allied professions or a strong volunteer program. The essence of good palliative care (and of all health care) should be what patients and their families have been telling us they want, over and over again in the literature. That is, that they want to be treated by people who are both competent and compassionate, and they want to be treated with dignity and respect.

In an article entitled "Dignity in the Terminally Ill: A Developing Empirical Model" (Chochinov et al. 2002, 434), the authors asked dying patients how they understood and defined the term "dignity." They found that terms such as "pride, self-respect, quality of life, well-being, hope, and self-esteem all overlap conceptually with the term dignity" (441), and their data supported the findings from another study, which concluded that "rather than viewing death with dignity as a separate construct, it might be viewed as an interactive process between the dying and their caretakers" (441).

Given this conclusion, how can one health care profession presume to take ownership of the art of treating the dying with respect and dignity? By Rachel Remen's definition of healing, aren't we all (including family members, volunteers, and friends) capable of being healers for those who are dying? What is lost when turf wars in health care take precedence over the need to provide compassionate, respectful care that starts with mutual respect for each other? How did we get to this place where it has become so important to defend our expertise, often at the expense of working together to offer healing to those who are in our care? We need to learn how to be as comfortable simply sitting with the questions that arise in the presence of death as we are in seeking explanations and answers After all, as Charles Lochner reminds us, "it is not that we have the answers that make us healers, but that we share the questions" (personal communication).

And so it will be the endless questions about life and death, some not even thought of yet much less voiced, that I will embrace and that will accompany me on my ongoing quest to find comfort and strength in my belief that "the quester cultivates the discipline of doubt . . . finds freedom in the unknowing" (Sam Keen 1994, 78).

I will continue to hope that as clinicians approach the bedsides of the dying in the course of their work, they will become willing to give up their reliance on labels to tell them who the person is before them, just as they are willing to relinquish their ownership of parts of the human experience, as if their expertise will ever be more important to those they serve than their humanity.

As for me, when I die, all that I need to be true is captured in Raymond Carver's last poem (1989) before his own death, and that is,

> To call myself beloved, to feel myself
> beloved on this earth.
> —Raymond Carver, "Late Fragment"

REFERENCES

Carver, R. 1989. *A new path to the waterfall.* New York: Atlantic Monthly.

Chochinov, H. M., T. Hack, S. McClement, L. Kristjanson, and M. Harlos. 2002. Dignity in the terminally ill: A developing empirical model. *Social Science & Medicine* 54: 433–43.

Kearney, M. 1996. *Mortally wounded.* New York: Scribner.

Keen, S. 1994. *Hymns to an unknown god.* New York: Bantam Books.

Kushner, H. 1983. *When bad things happen to good people.* New York: Avon Books.

Muller, W. 1996. *How then shall we live?* New York: Bantam Books.

Nepo, M. 2006. http://www.marknepo.com/books/unlearning.htm.

Oliver, M. 2003. In blackwater woods. *Risking everything: 110 poems of love and revelation.* ed. R. Housden. New York: Harmony Books, 72–73.

Remen, R. 1997. *Kitchen table wisdom.* New York: Riverhead Books.

Rolling, J. H. 2004. Searching self-image: Identities to be self-evident. *Qualitative Inquiry* 10(6): 869–84.

CHAPTER 8

Final Reflections on Spirituality in Hospice Palliative Care

PAUL BRAMADAT AND KELLI I. STAJDUHAR

As MANY READERS WILL KNOW, the present volume seeks to address specific problems and questions that arose out of the earlier volume in this series, *Religious Understandings of a Good Death in Hospice Palliative Care*. In particular, the authors of that volume reflected on the considerations that hospice palliative caregivers (and others) ought to bear in mind when engaging with Jews, Christians, Hindus, Muslims, and others during the final stages of life. For people who think of themselves and their deaths in formally religious terms, it is of great importance that our health care systems as well as our broader communities respond sensitively and knowledgably to explicitly religious requirements; to fail to do so, in fact, would demonstrate an appalling disregard for the integrity and autonomy of these people at a time in their lives when they are most in need of informed compassion and solidarity.

Nevertheless, while formal religious requirements related to death and dying are central concerns of millions of people, "spirituality" is rapidly eclipsing "religion" as the concept that prevails as hospice staff work with patients at the end of life. This change has not emerged in a vacuum, of course; in other contexts in our society, similar processes are at work. In the present volume, we gathered authors who we felt could reflect critically on the implications of the ascendancy of the concept of "spirituality" in hospice palliative care. Instead of recapitulating the findings of each of the chapters, in our conclusion we would like to reflect on some of the key lessons we have learned during our research and the most fruitful areas of future investigation.

OUR MAIN FINDINGS

The first issue we faced—as individual authors as well as a team—was the establishment of an operational definition of the concept of "spirituality." Even though the definition of "religion" is debated by scholars of religious studies, it is clear that in general parlance, both among hospice palliative care clinicians and certainly in the nursing and medical literatures, religion is now defined mostly in terms of its doctrinal, institutional, legal, ritual, prescriptive and proscriptive, authoritarian, objective, and historical features. That is, when most people think of religion—whether they are facing the end of their lives or simply reflecting on the term in general—they think in terms of formal structures that create order, laws, customs, and meaning.

A comprehensive history of what happened to the traditional power of religion in the last 150 years in Western societies is beyond the scope of this project (see Taylor 2007), but it is worthwhile to remember that the twentieth and twenty-first centuries are famous for their crises of faith, creating doubts that have crept into many lives and that have undermined the once firm relationships between Western societies and religion. The intellectual forebears of these crises are, of course, Freud, Marx, Weber, Nietzsche, Darwin, higher biblical criticism, and more recently radical (or "the new") atheists such as Christopher Hitchens and Richard Dawkins; the historical forebears are notably the horrors of Auschwitz, and the "killing fields" of Cambodia, and more recently the events of September 11th; the political and philosophical forebears are the feminist and civil rights movements and postmodernism. Other sources of ferment and tumult exist, of course, but the point is simply that today, both in the health care and political arenas, religion is no longer generally assumed—if it ever had been—to be a generally unproblematic social good. Indeed, throughout the West, the formal and informal privileges once granted solely to Christianity are either being extricated in favor of a putatively "neutral" public sphere or extended to the benefit of non-Christian citizens of multicultural societies.

In response, spirituality has rushed in to fill the void created by the "problematization" of religion. But how shall we speak of spirituality? Measure it? Evaluate it—empirically and morally? Several of the chapters of this book explore the problem with the definition of this now central term in hospice palliative care (and throughout the nursing and medical literatures); many of the authors reflect on the challenges facing natural and social scientists and health scientists wanting to critically examine the reasons that spirituality is framed as a more attractive, neutral, and inclusive concept than religion. One of the problems is that spirituality as a term and concept is both new and old: while there are, for example, traditions of Hindu and Christian spirituality that have been in use for thousands of years, there is something also quite new about the term as it has assumed such a prominent role (in roughly the last twenty or thirty years at most) in the relevant literatures and clinical settings featured in this book.

Many of the chapters outline the sometimes contradictory features of the term: in some cases it refers to antireligious individualized spiritual inklings, and in other cases, it refers to personal moments of transcendence experienced firmly within a formal religious context. Spirituality is usually defined as or associated with an openness to nondogmatic and extra-institutional wisdom related to human suffering and well-being, an abiding interest in a personal experience of transcendence that fosters dignity and acceptance, and a common commitment to being or feeling "at one" with the universe or the planet. Moreover, it is often defined as an important means of correcting the narrowly biomedical focus on strictly physical maladies that is thought to typify Western health care; as such, attention to spirituality by care providers can complement the treatments patients are offered: these treatments evolve from merely biomedical or at most biopsychosocial to biopsychosocial-spiritual (see chapter 3 by Bramadat and Kaufert). In this sense,

a concern for the spiritual needs of patients in hospice palliative care supposedly enables caregivers to treat each individual
more comprehensively than would be possible within a strictly
biomedical model. Of course, this is itself a contestable claim,
and it reflects an assumption that, as Garces-Foley observes,
excludes many people who wish to turn to formal religions
rather than spirituality during this period in their lives. Nevertheless, most of the chapters (see the chapters by Wilson, Sinclair and Chochinov, and Bruce and Stajduhar) observe that
attention to spirituality is generally considered by hospice palliative care staff to be a boon to the mental and physical health
of the patients and families involved in hospice palliative care.

The second issue that is evident in a number of chapters is
the lingering power of the biomedical model throughout the
health care arena. As we saw in both the first and the present volume, such power is evident in the defunding of spiritual care (sometimes still called chaplaincy) departments when
health systems face budget cuts. Such power is also apparent in
the desire among some in the hospice palliative care field and
beyond to boil down complex human spiritual traditions and
phenomena into simple guidelines and measures that staff can
consult when dealing with particular kinds of adherents. While
such guidelines promote an efficient model of patient care and
may provide important tools for guiding clinical decision making, we must also consider the implications of using standardized instruments to assess what is an inherently complex issue.
It may well be more helpful for care providers working with the
dying to have a general orientation to, for example, Hindu and
Christian principles and requirements associated with death. If
the diversity within Hinduism and Christianity makes simple
checklists of extremely limited use for these populations, the
diversity within what we loosely called the SBNR (spiritual but
not religious) cohort makes such shortcuts utterly futile. Nonetheless, the commitment to efficiency within the health care
system as a whole creates a pressure on hospice palliative care
providers to systematize that which is by definition unsystem-
atic—the spiritual sensibilities of a cohort that either eschews
or creatively recombines traditional categories. As we see in the
chapter on spirituality care in nursing by Bruce and Stajduhar,

assumptions that every dying person has a spiritual dimension that can be assessed, measured, and treated or that considerations of spirituality and spiritual distress require a nursing "diagnosis" can potentially negate and make invisible the individuality of the dying person. Moreover, nursing's preoccupation with finding a consensus on the definition of spirituality and on operationalizing and measuring the concept has in some ways limited conversations of how to practically provide care to patients that have spiritual concerns.

In medicine, the power of the "hidden curriculum" apparent in medical schools and residency training programs also demonstrates the dominance of the biomedical model. As Bramadat and Kaufert explain, many educators promote medical humanities and bioethics programs that generally frame religion and spirituality quite positively as integral features of patients' lives and experiences of suffering and death, and thus as worthy of physicians' attention. However, these same programs generally do not require medical students and residents to prove what one might call their "religious literacy" on examinations, and in practice instructors avoid case studies that might require student physicians to pay close attention to the effects of religious and spiritual ideation and practice. As such, these programs tend—perhaps unintentionally—to undermine some of the insights we have discussed here about the ubiquity and efficacy of the concept of spirituality (and the value of religious or spiritual literacy among staff) and tend to remind us of the concentration of power within the allopathic medical establishment.

FUTURE LINES OF INQUIRY

One of the most pressing needs not just in the field of religion and health but indeed in the study of contemporary religious phenomena more generally is continued examination of the spiritual but not religious cohort. Most religious studies scholars recognize the implied shift as a fairly identifiable sociological phenomenon, and certainly colleagues in the medical, nursing, educational, and social services fields confirm anecdotally that the shift from talking about religion to talking about spirituality is especially evident among people under forty. However, it became clear at our team meetings that even among those whose chapters dealt explicitly with this group of people in a single health care setting, there are disagreements about how to define the phenomenon, how large the cohort can be said to be, how profound are its ramifications for traditional religions, and how SBNR people might be distinguished from SDNR (spiritual and definitely not religious) people. At present, research into the nature of the SBNR cohort is in its infancy. As such, in order to understand better the implications in the shift from focusing on religion to focusing on spirituality—not just in hospice palliative care but throughout health care in general—we need to have more thorough analyses of the SBNR phenomenon itself. Related to this issue, the discursive shift that we see in both the literature and the practice of hospice palliative care with its increasing emphasis on "spiritual care" and a minimization of the role of religion will have implications for patients and families that need to be analyzed in greater depth. For example, how do these shifts within institutional contexts, from religion to spirituality, influence the ways in which dying people and their families are cared for? How do providers respond to these shifts and how might these shifts influence their care of the dying? How do provider beliefs, values, and spiritual or religious traditions influence the ways in which they approach the people they care for and about?

Much of the research on spirituality in hospice palliative care has focused on conceptualizations of spirituality, on developing guidelines and measures to assess spiritual needs, on "treating" spiritual distress, and on understanding patient experiences. Many of the chapters in this volume reflect these emphases along with a concurrent concern regarding funding cuts to spiritual care programs within health care institutions. While hospice palliative care has in general, and historically, valued and provided spiritual care more effectively than other areas of health care, such programs are often threatened by funding cuts. Financial pressures on health care institutions force scholars and practitioners to consider new ways of explaining how we might provide spiritual support to the dying. Action-oriented research into ways of integrating existing spiritual support systems into health care systems may create innovative models of care delivery. Research has shown that existential, spiritual, and traditional religious issues are of great importance to dying individuals and their families, and so defining how such support can be made available would be important.

The challenges of defining, operationalizing, and measuring spirituality or spiritual "distress" have been well articulated in this volume; many of its authors have questioned the assumed wisdom of these efforts. While it is clear that having an understanding of the concept of spirituality might be useful in the provision of care at the end of life, clinicians would be well advised to ask themselves several questions: What is it that leads those of us in the health professions to search for a singular definition of spirituality? What are the implications of uncritically implementing spiritual care guidelines in populations that are inherently diverse in their belief systems and values? While there may be value in our continued efforts to excavate a concept that has eluded definition, we ought to do so with a critical and humble mind, attempting to unpack and problematize the underlying assumptions that guide our efforts, and resisting tidy and likely unintentionally alienating definitions of the concept.

Finally, we see in both the first and present volume that conflicts can emerge between dying individuals and families and health care providers when there is a lack of understanding, or even intolerance for particular spiritual or religious beliefs and rituals. Anecdotally we know that conflicts arise (see Will, chapter 5), but there is little evidence to help us understand how common these conflicts are and why they occur. Such understanding could enhance respectful and compassionate care at the end of life.

WHAT ARE THE PRACTICAL
IMPLICATIONS OF THIS PROJECT?

In several of the chapters in this book—though most notably in the chapters on nursing and chaplaincy—authors have emphasized the importance of listening. This may well seem like a bland prescription that would be worthwhile for anyone to consider, but it is in fact the best means available for responding meaningfully when the concept of spirituality is invoked by clinicians, patients, and their families. As mentioned earlier, and as especially evident in the chapters by Grant and Causton, there can be no simple way to respond to someone whose approach to the end of life falls outside of the boundaries of formal religion. However, as several authors have argued, a posture of openness, curiosity, and humility will go a long way to avoiding alienating the people involved. Causton encourages people to adopt the approach of fellow "explorers" rather than "detectives."

These two metaphors are quite instructive. The detective role is, of course, indicative of the more formal efficiency-oriented "check-box" model, according to which a hospice palliative care staff member would approach a patient and pose some questions to determine—as a detective might—what a person's formal religious affiliations or spiritual needs might be. Again, such inquiries no doubt aim to provide the best possible care for the patient. However, people whose spiritual lives have developed outside of a singular traditional religious framework, perhaps over many decades, may well be expected to resist or resent any efforts to be fitted into a tidy category. A more sensitive, sensible, and ultimately more effective way to approach such people would be to listen at some considerable length to their stories about their spiritual life and the ways they are framing their own deaths. If patients feel clinicians are willing to explore a set of questions, even an inchoate series of hunches and concerns, they will likely be more able to trust that they are being seen as a whole person rather than merely as exemplifications of medical breakdowns. This approach would certainly be consistent with what Dame Cicely Saunders originally intended when she founded the modern hospice movement.

Listening is easier said than done, however. If clinicians and others in the support network of the patient are going to attend more deliberately to an individual as he or she reflects on the spiritual dimensions of his or her mortality, it would be ideal if in fact there was some kind of base of knowledge shared by both. It would not be very unusual, for example, for a single patient's spiritual musings to include references to

Buddhism, Christianity, and Aboriginal spirituality. If the clinician is not merely going to act as a detective, waiting until the patient indicates that she or he is an adherent of a particular religious tradition, then the clinician—now reframed as the fellow explorer—would presumably need some basic familiarity with the core sensibilities of each of these perspectives.

Unfortunately, our society is marked by the ascendancy of a form of secularism that often discourages even factual and dispassionate discussions about religion. This particular ideological perspective has arguably produced a fairly widespread "religious illiteracy." In particular many public educational systems are so concerned about the challenges of providing balanced education about religion that they often exclude it from curricula altogether (Seljak 2005). This is problematic because even highly idiosyncratic spiritualities that are increasingly likely to be articulated in hospice palliative care contexts often combine elements of existing religious traditions. As such, we recommend the explicit inclusion of religion and spirituality as central topics in the training of hospice palliative care clinicians, and health care providers more generally. This may come in the form of enhanced humanities courses for nurses, physicians, social workers, and other health professionals, or in ongoing professional development activities. As well, it will be important to include in such training opportunities for clinicians to reflect openly not only on their own values, beliefs, and assumptions but on how these might influence the provision of spiritual care for dying people.

It is quite clear that there has been an ascendancy of spirituality coupled with a concomitant retreat of the concept of religion in academic and clinical discussions related to Western hospice palliative care. As we have outlined in this book, clinicians and scholars interested in this transition, and in the ongoing development of their field, face serious challenges. However, their common interest in the compassionate care of the dying should guide them toward an effective approach to this relatively new phenomenon. Such efforts are surely in keeping with the deep moral impulse that gave birth to the hospice movement so many decades ago.

REFERENCES

Seljak, D. 2005. Education, multiculturalism, and religion. In *Religion and ethnicity in Canada*, ed. P. Bramadat and D. Seljak. Toronto: Pearson Education Canada, 178–200.

Taylor, C. 2007. *The secular age*. Boston: Harvard University Press.

Contributors

PAUL BRAMADAT is Associate Professor of Religious Studies and Director of the Centre for Studies in Religion and Society at the University of Victoria. He has published broadly on issues related to religious and ethnic diversity in Canada and globally. He is the author of *The Church on the World's Turf: An Evangelical Christian Group at a Secular University* (Oxford, 2000) and editor, with Mathias Koenig, of *International Migration and the Governance of Religious Diversity* (2009) and, with David Seljak, *Christianity and Ethnicity in Canada* (2008). He is currently at work on several new initiatives including a study of religiously affiliated immigrant settlement agencies in British Columbia, an edited volume on security and state responses to religious radicalization, and a project examining religious and cultural roots of vaccine refusal.

ANNE BRUCE is Associate Professor in the School of Nursing at the University of Victoria. She received her PhD from the University of British Columbia in 2002. Her research interests include existential suffering in end of life, Buddhist approaches to hospice palliative care, contemplative practices in nursing, and interpretive and narrative research methodologies.

ELIZABETH CAUSTON has a master's degree in social work. She has worked in the social work field for over forty years, including fourteen years at the Victoria Hospice in Victoria, BC, on the Palliative Response Team. Now retired, she continues to teach workshops across Canada and online on a variety of topics related to psychosocial and communication issues for nurses, community health workers, physicians, and other health professionals. She is also working with a research team at the University of Victoria exploring ways to improve palliative care across all health care settings.

HARVEY MAX CHOCHINOV is Distinguished Professor of Psychiatry at the University of Manitoba and Director of the Manitoba Palliative Care Research Unit, CancerCare Manitoba. He holds the only Canada Research Chair in Palliative Care and is a member of the Governing Council of the Canadian Institutes of Health Research. He also chairs the CIHR's Standing Committee on Ethics. His research has covered a broad range of issues pertaining to palliative care, including depression, desire for death, will to live, and dignity at the end of life. He is a recipient of the Queen's Golden Jubilee Medal and the Order of Manitoba; he is the founder and chair of the Canadian Virtual Hospice, a fellow of the Royal Society of Canada, and a fellow of the Canadian Academy of Health Sciences.

HAROLD COWARD is Professor Emeritus of History and founding director of the Centre for Studies in Religion and Society at the University of Victoria. He is the author and editor of several books, including *A Cross-Cultural Dialogue on Health Care Ethics*, *Religious Understandings of a Good Death in Hospice Palliative Care*, and *The Perfectibility of Human Nature in Eastern and Western Thought*.

KATHLEEN GARCES-FOLEY is Associate Professor of Religious Studies at Marymount University, specializing in contemporary American religious life. Her research interests include funeral practices, immigration, young adults, and multiracial churches. She is the author of *Crossing the Ethnic Divide: The Multiethnic Church on a Mission* and editor of *Death and Religion in a Changing World*.

PATRICK GRANT is Professor Emeritus, University of Victoria, British Columbia, Canada. He was educated at the Queen's

University of Belfast and at Sussex University. In 1990 he was elected Fellow of the Royal Society of Canada. He is the author of numerous books, including a trilogy on literature and the idea of the person. Other titles deal with the New Testament as literature, Western mysticism, literary Modernism, the scientific revolution, and the literature and culture of the English Renaissance. He has written three books on religion and ethnic conflict. Two of these are on modern Northern Ireland and one is on modern Sri Lanka.

JOSEPH KAUFERT is Professor in the Department of Community Health Sciences and the Centre for Aboriginal Health Research in the Faculty of Medicine at the University of Manitoba. His areas of research concentration are in the fields of medical anthropology, disability studies, clinical and research ethics, and Indigenous health. His research with urban First Nations and Inuit communities has documented the impact of language interpreters and cultural advocates in urban hospitals. His current research involves exploring the impact of cultural and structural factors in ethical frameworks for informed consent and end-of-life decision making. He is currently coprincipal investigator in two CIHR funded research projects documenting 1) ethical dimensions and barriers to compassionate end-of-life care for persons made vulnerable: and 2) the ethical dimension of the participation of human subjects in health research.

SHANE SINCLAIR is a Canadian Institutes of Health Research postdoctoral fellow in the Manitoba Palliative Care Research Unit at the University of Manitoba in Winnipeg. He is also the Spiritual Care Coordinator at the Tom Baker Cancer Centre in Calgary, where he holds an appointment in the Faculty of Medicine, Department of Oncology, Division of Palliative Medicine at the University of Calgary. His PhD dissertation, focused on the spirituality of palliative care professionals in Canada, was nominated for the Governor General's Gold Medal Award. He is a board-certified chaplain with the Canadian Association for Spiritual Care and has provided spiritual care in the areas of palliative care and oncology over the past decade.

KELLI I. STAJDUHAR is Associate Professor in the School of Nursing and Centre on Aging at the University of Victoria. She has worked in oncology, palliative care, and gerontology for over twenty years as a staff nurse, nurse clinician, clinical nurse specialist, and academic. Her clinical research has focused on health service needs for those at the end of life and their families and on the needs of marginalized and vulnerable populations, particularly seniors, patients with HIV/AIDS, and injection-drug-using populations. Dr. Stajduhar holds a New Investigator Award from the Canadian Institutes of Health Research and a Scholar Award from the Michael Smith Foundation for Health Research.

W. WILSON WILL III is the inaugural Medical Humanities Postdoctoral Fellow at the Humanities Research Center at Rice University. He received his PhD in medical anthropology and social studies of medicine from McGill University in 2010. His dissertation explores the training and work of hospital chaplains through an analysis of the epistemological and narrative interactions of religion and biomedicine. Current research projects include the clinical interactions of multiple types of hope, the relationship between statistics and theology, and the notion of the biomedicalization of American religion.

Index